Contents

KU-183-062

OXFORD ONCOLOGY LIBRARY

Systemic Treatment of Prostate Cancer

Edited by

Prof. Alan Horwich

Institute of Cancer Research
and Royal Marsden NHS Foundation Trust,
Sutton, UK

University of Nottingham
at Derby Library

OXFORD
UNIVERSITY PRESS

OXFORD
UNIVERSITY PRESS

Great Clarendon Street, Oxford OX2 6DP

Oxford University Press is a department of the University of Oxford.
It furthers the University's objective of excellence in research, scholarship,
and education by publishing worldwide in

Oxford New York

Auckland Cape Town Dar es Salaam Hong Kong Karachi
Kuala Lumpur Madrid Melbourne Mexico City Nairobi
New Delhi Shanghai Taipei Toronto

With offices in

Argentina Austria Brazil Chile Czech Republic France Greece
Guatemala Hungary Italy Japan Poland Portugal Singapore
South Korea Switzerland Thailand Turkey Ukraine Vietnam

Oxford is a registered trade mark of Oxford University Press
in the UK and in certain other countries

Published in the United States
by Oxford University Press Inc., New York

© Oxford University Press, 2010

The moral rights of the author(s) have been asserted
Database right Oxford University Press (maker)

First published 2010

All rights reserved. No part of this publication may be reproduced,
stored in a retrieval system, or transmitted, in any form or by any means,
without the prior permission in writing of Oxford University Press,
or as expressly permitted by law, or under terms agreed with the appropriate
reprographics rights organization. Enquiries concerning reproduction
outside the scope of the above should be sent to the Rights Department,
Oxford University Press, at the address above

You must not circulate this book in any other binding or cover
and you must impose the same condition on any acquirer

British Library Cataloguing in Publication Data

Data available

Library of Congress Cataloging in Publication Data

Data available

Typeset by Newgen Imaging Systems (P) Ltd., Chennai, India
Printed in Great Britain
on acid-free paper by
Ashford Colour Press Ltd., Gosport, Hampshire.

ISBN 978–0–19–956142–1

10 9 8 7 6 5 4 3 2 1

1006572667

Preface

Prostate cancer requires systemic management in a number of contexts, including adjuvant treatment, biochemical (PSA) relapse, asymptomatic metastasis, and palliation of distressing problems such as bone pain, spinal cord compression and lymphoedema. Technologies presented include hormone therapies, bone-seeking isotopes, bisphosphonates, cytotoxic drugs, and biologically-targeted drugs in development, and the emphasis has been to provide the clinical evidence underpinning appropriate treatment choice since this can both relieve symptoms and prolong life. Patients with metastatic disease usually live for several years, and in contrast to other cancers, it is common that patients gain from active treatment even of third and fourth relapse.

In producing this handbook, it has been a pleasure to work with authoritative contributors with such extensive and close experience of caring for patients with prostate cancer. We share the hope that it will help to guide physicians with the challenging responsibility of providing rational advice, and the book is dedicated particularly to those patients whose participation in clinical trials has enabled the principles of management to be established.

Symbols and abbreviations

AA	Anti-androgen
ADT	Androgen deprivation therapy
AR	Androgen receptor
ASCO	American Society of Clinical Oncology
BCR	Biochemical recurrence
BFGF	Basic fibroblast growth factors
CAB	Combined androgen blockade
CML	Chronic myeloid leukemia
CPA	Cyproterone acetate
CRPC	Castration-resistant prostate cancer
CSDX	Casodex®
CTC	Circulating tumor cells
DES	Diethylstilbestrol
DHT	5α-dihydrotestosterone
EDTMP	Ethylenediaminetetramethylene phosphonic acid
EGF	Epidermal growth factor
EMP	Estramustine phosphate
EPCP	Early Prostate Cancer Programme
EORTC	European Organisation for Research and Treatment of Cancer
ERBT	External beam radiotherapy
FDA	Food and Drug Administration
GnRH	Gonadotropin-releasing hormone
HEDP	Hydroxyethylene diphosphonate
HPG	Hypothalamic-pituitary-gonadal
HSP	Heat shock proteins
IGF-I	Insulin-like growth factor-I
IL-6	Interleukin-6
KGF	Keratinocyte growth factor
LH	Luteinizing hormone
LHRH	Luteinizing hormone releasing hormone

MAPK	Mitogen activated protein kinase
MRC	Medical Research Council
NICE	National Institute for Health and Clinical Excellence
PCTCG	Prostate Cancer Trialists' Collaborative Group
PCWG	Prostate Cancer Working Group
PDGF	Platelet derived growth factors
PKA	Protein kinase A
PKC	Protein kinase C
PPI	present pain intensity
PSA	Prostate specific antigen
PSADT	PSA doubling time
SPARC	Satraplatin and Prednisone Against Refractory Cancer
SRE	Skeletal related event
SSRI	Selective serotonin reuptake inhibitors
SWOG	Southwest Oncology Group
VEGF	Vascular endothelial growth factor

Contributors

Ajjai S Alva
Division of Hematology-Oncology
Department of Internal Medicine
University of Michigan
Ann Arbor, Michigan
USA

Lionel L. Bañez
Assistant Professor
Division of Urologic Surgery
Duke University Medical Center
Durham, NC
USA

Johann DeBono
Senior Lecturer and
Consultant in Oncology
Section of Medicine
Institute of Cancer Research
Royal Marsden Hospital
Drug Development Unit
Sutton, UK

David P Dearnaley
Professor of Urological Oncology
The Royal Marsden Hospital and
Institute of Cancer Research
Sutton, UK

Sophie Fossa
Departments of Clinical
Radiotherapy and Oncology
The Norwegian Radium Hospital
University of Oslo
Oslo, Norway

Karim Fizazi
Head of the Department
of Medicine and
Chairman of the GU
Oncology Group
Institut Gustave Roussy
Villejuif, France

Stephen Freedland
Associate Professor of Urology
and Pathology,
and Director of Outcomes and
Translational Research
Urological Surgery
Duke University Medical
Center
Durham, North Carolina
USA

Marine Gross-Goupil
Institut Gustave Roussy
Villejuif, France

Alan Horwich
Professor of Radiotherapy
The Royal Marsden Hospital and
Institute of Cancer Research
Sutton, UK

Maha Hussain
Professor of Medicine and Urology
University of Michigan
Comprehensive Cancer Center
Ann Arbor, Michigan
USA

Wolfgang Lilleby
Head of Urooncology and
Radiation Oncologist
The Norwegian Radium
Hospital
University of Oslo
Oslo, Norway

Yohann Loriot
Institut Gustave Roussy
Villejuif, France

xi

Malcolm D Mason
Professor and Head of
Urooncology and Radiation
Oncologist
Cardiff University
School of Medicine
Velindre Hospital
Cardiff, UK

Danish Mazhar
Consultant Medical Oncologist
Addenbrooke's Hospital
Cambridge

Daniel M. Moreira
Postdoctoral Associate
Division of Urologic Surgery
Duke University Medical Center
Durham, NC
USA

Judd W. Moul
Chief, Division of Urologic Surgery
Duke University Medical Center
Durham, NC
USA

Christopher C Parker
Consultant in Oncology
The Royal Marsden Hospital and
Institute of Cancer Research
Sutton, UK

Shahneen Sandhu
Clinical Research Fellow
The Royal Marsden Hospital and
Institute of Cancer Research
Drug Development Unit
Sutton, UK

Mike D Shelley
Principal Clinical Research
Scientist
Head of the Cochrane Urological
Cancers Unit
Research Department,
Velindre NHS Trust Hospital,
Cardiff, UK.

Guru Sonpavde
Urologic Oncology Program
Texas Oncology
Veterans Affairs Medical Center,
Baylor College of Medicine
Houston, Texas
USA

Cora N.Sternberg
San Camillo and
Forlanini Hospitals
Nuovi Padiglione IV
Rome, Italy

Jonathan H Waxman
Professor of Medical Oncology
and Consultant in Oncology
Imperial College London
London, UK

xii

Chapter 1

Biological principles of hormone therapy

Danish Mazhar and Jonathan Waxman

Key points

- Androgen receptor (AR) signalling is necessary for the development of prostate cancer
- Androgens exert their biological effects through AR
- Androgen-deprivation therapy for prostate cancer was described over 50 years ago and remains the mainstay of systemic therapy
- Although the mechanisms by which prostate cancer cells change androgen sensitivity are unclear, it is believed that the tumour cells must either bypass or adapt the AR-mediated cell growth pathway in order to survive in a low androgen microenvironment during androgen ablation therapy
- With increasing understanding of the genes and pathways that drive castration-refratory prostate cancer, therapeutic agents are being developed that act on the key molecular targets.

1.1 Introduction

Prostate cancer, along with breast cancer, represents a paradigm of hormone-sensitive malignancy. The importance of androgens and androgen receptor (AR) in primary prostate cancer is now well-established. Locally advanced and metastatic disease is usually treated with androgen ablation, which is an effective form of therapy but only for a limited amount of time. When the disease has become hormone refractory, or castration refractory, then it is more challenging to manage. The role of AR in prostate cancers that recur despite androgen ablation therapy is still not clear. Most of these tumours express prostate specific antigen (PSA), an androgen-regulated gene; moreover, AR is generally highly expressed in recurrent prostate cancer. It is proposed that AR continues to play a role in many of these tumours and that it is not only the levels of AR, ligands, and co-regulators, but also changes in cell signalling that induce AR action in recurrent prostate cancer. These pathways are, therefore, potential targets for future therapeutic approaches.

This chapter discusses the principles of biological treatment in the management of prostate cancer, including the rationales for further hormone manipulations in those whose disease becomes castration refractory.

1.2 **Physiological functions of androgens**

Androgens are lipophilic steroids that are required for the development of the male sex organs and secondary sexual characteristics. The prostate gland is dependent on androgen stimulation for its development and differentiation. After about 8 weeks of fetal development, the fetal testes initiate synthesis of testosterone, which is converted by the enzyme 5α-reductase, to the more active androgen, 5α-dihydrotestosterone (DHT). Both DHT and testosterone bind to intracellular AR in the reproductive tract, resulting in development and differentiation of the prostate and of male internal and external genitalia. After initial development, these structures undergo little further growth during the remainder of fetal life and childhood, but a surge in testosterone secretion by the testes at puberty and a consequent surge in DHT, results in their further growth and maturation into functional adult sexual organs. Although androgens are principally synthesized by the testes, with production stimulated by luteinizing hormone (LH), they are also secreted by the adrenal cortex, ovaries and other organs in small amounts.

The prostate is dependent on androgens for functioning throughout adult life. Over 90% of testosterone in the prostate is converted into DHT. This occurs mostly in stromal cells, after which DHT is transported to the epithelium. Benign prostatic hyperplasia is a common condition, evident in up to 90% of men by 80 years of age, caused by proliferation of epithelial and stromal cells. Without androgens, the prostate undergoes significant atrophy.

1.3 **AR and its role in prostate cancer**

Prostate adenocarcinoma has recently become the most prevalent male malignancy in industrialized nations and the second leading cause of cancer-related mortality (10,000 per annum in the UK). The incidence is 35,000 per year in the UK where the average lifetime risk of a man developing prostate cancer is around 1 in 13.

Prostate cancer incidence increases exponentially with age and many men will not develop the disease until they are over 70 years.

Huggins and Hodges in the early 1940s first observed the androgen-dependency of prostate cancer. It is now established that prostate cancer development and progression is dependent on testosterone and DHT and the effects of these androgens on cell proliferation and differentiation are mediated through AR. AR is expressed in virtually all prostate cancers, including metastatic disease and those refractory to therapy.

During embryogenesis, AR is expressed in mesenchymal cells of the urogenital sinus, with subsequent temporal expression in epithelial cells. The adult human prostate consists of epithelial and stromal tissues and both cellular components express AR. Androgen treatment leads to a rapid decrease in AR mRNA. However it also stabilizes the protein, with the overall effect of increasing AR protein levels in the prostate. This differential regulation is unique to the prostate. For example, the effect of androgen stimulation in bone is to increase both AR mRNA and AR protein levels. Activation of AR by androgens in the normal prostate regulates proliferation of prostate cells by inducing expression of key cell cycle regulators such as the cyclin-dependent kinases (cdks) cdk2 and cdk4. Androgens also stimulate secretory responses and synthesis of important prostatic lipids. Activation of AR by androgens also drives the expression of prostate-specific antigen (PSA), a serine protease produced by the prostate gland at very high concentrations. Serum levels of PSA are increased in prostate cancer as well as in prostatic inflammatory conditions and benign prostatic hyperplasia.

Androgen-independent pathways are also known to regulate AR activity in prostate cells. For example, in the absence of androgen, phosphorylation of residues contained within the ligand-independent activation function (AF-1) in the N-terminal region of the AR protein leads to ligand-independent activation. Also, several growth factors have been shown to cause AR activation through stimulation of second-messenger pathways. Insulin-like growth factor-I (IGF-I), keratinocyte growth factor (KGF), epidermal growth factor (EGF) and vascular endothelial growth factor (VEGF) all stimulate hormone-independent activation of AR. AR can be directly activated by substances that increase protein kinase A (PKA) and protein kinase C (PKC) activities. Additionally, interleukin-6 (IL-6) has been shown to activate AR in the absence of androgens via pathways dependent on increased phosphorylation of mitogen activated protein kinase (MAPK) and PKC. Thus, even in the presence of androgen ablation therapies, AR may be activated by growth factors, interleukins and kinases, stimulating tumour growth and contributing to the development of hormone-refractory disease.

3

1.4 **Endocrine therapy for prostate cancer**

Whilst localized prostate cancer can potentially be cured by surgery or radical radiotherapy, many patients present late, after the disease has become advanced or has metastasized. Hormonal treatment is generally indicated in patients with locally advanced or metastatic prostate cancer, or in the setting of relapsed disease.

Until around a decade ago, the standard endocrine treatment for prostate cancer was surgical castration, or administration of the female hormones, estrogen or medroxyprogesterone acetate, to inhibit androgen-regulated tumour growth. However, side-effects of estrogen therapies include development of secondary female sexual characteristics (e.g., breast development), venous and arterial thrombosis, nausea, loss of libido and impotence. Today, initial hormone therapy may involve suppression of the hypothalamus-pituitary-gonadal axis, using luteinizing hormone releasing hormone (LHRH) analogues, such as leuprorelin and goserelin. These long-acting peptide analogues of LHRH agonists produce an initial stimulation of LH and FSH secretion by the pituitary gland. However, a negative feedback results in a long-term down-regulation of gonadotrophin release from the pituitary and a block in testosterone production by the testes. Side-effects include impotence, anaemia, osteoporosis, mild reduction in muscle tone and hot flushes.

The strategy of complete androgen withdrawal by coupling surgical or chemical castration with anti-androgen treatment may produce superior therapeutic efficacy, as discussed in chapter 5. Orchidectomy leads to the removal of testicular androgens, but does not affect production of circulating androgens, such as dehydroepiandrosterone and androstenedione from the adrenal glands. Though weak AR agonists themselves, these chemicals can be converted into testosterone by intra-prostatic enzymes. Clinical studies in the early 1980s led to the notion that these adrenal androgens play an important role in progression of prostate cancers and hence the concept of combined blockade of both androgen production and inhibition of AR function to produce complete androgen withdrawal was adopted. This has encouraged the use of the so-called anti-androgen drugs, including the mixed agonist/antagonist, cyproterone acetate (CPA) which had already been introduced in the 1970s, and the pure, non-steroidal anti-androgen, bicalutamide or Casodex®. These drugs bind to AR to prevent its activation block and are used in combination with chemical or surgical castration.

1.5 Resistance to endocrine therapy in prostate cancer

Current endocrine treatment for prostate cancer is limited by the development of resistance, as the surviving tumour cells lose their dependency on androgens for growth and proliferate in the absence of serum androgens. In the past, this was erroneously believed to be due to outgrowth of AR-negative tumour cells or down-regulation of AR expression. As yet, the molecular mechanisms underlying the acquisition of androgen-independent growth in the continuing presence of AR have not been defined, but potential mechanisms include mutation of the AR gene resulting in promiscuous ligand binding, activation of AR by other endocrine or paracrine growth factors independent of ligand binding, and AR gene amplification.

Studies in prostate cancer cell lines have shown that after long-term androgen withdrawal, levels of AR mRNA and protein gradually increase and that AR becomes acutely sensitive to even small amounts of androgen. Thus, the beneficial effects of androgen ablation are probably restricted to a limited time frame.

Point mutations of AR have not been frequently described in primary prostate cancers. However, a number of studies have shown that there is a high frequency of AR point mutations in metastatic lesions. The first AR point mutation was described in LNCaP, a cell line derived from a lymph node metastasis of a therapy-refractory prostate cancer. The point mutation substitutes an alanine for a threonine at position 877 and produces a mutant receptor with increased binding affinity for estrogen and progesterone. A number of single, or multiple point mutations in AR in prostate tumours and metastases have now been identified that lead to promiscuous activation of the receptor by binding of other steroid hormones, or even androgen antagonists, and may lead to accelerated progression of prostate cancer.

Activation of AR by non-steroidal hormones, such as growth factors, via the ligand-independent AF-1 of the receptor may also play a role in the development of resistance to anti-androgen therapies. Like many other steroid receptors, wild-type AR is involved in cross-talk with various growth factor signalling pathways as well as neurotransmitters and peptide hormones, many of which activate the receptor via the MAPK pathway. Studies have demonstrated that these substances are capable of potentiating the androgen-dependent activation of AR on a background of low androgen concentration, which may partly account for the relapse of patients with advanced prostate cancer. However, it is important to note that several of the non-steroidal anti-androgens, such as bicalutamide, inhibit ligand-independent activation of AR and therefore may be useful as a second line therapy after failure of steroidal anti-androgens such as CPA.

Further reading

Culig Z, Hobisch A, Bartsch G, and Klocker H (2000). Expression and function of androgen receptor in carcinoma of the prostate. *Microsc Res Tech*, **51**, 447–55.

Culig, Z, Hoffmann, J, Erdel, M, Eder, IE, Hobisch, A, Hittmair, A, Bartsch, G, Utermann, G, Schneider, MR, Parczyk, K, and Klocker, H (1999). Switch from antagonist to agonist of the androgen receptor bicalutamide is associated with prostate tumour progression in a new model system. *Br J Cancer*, **81**, 242–51.

Mendelsohn, LG (2000). Prostate cancer and the androgen receptor: strategies for the development of novel therapeutics. *Prog Drug Res*, **55**, 213–33.

Montgomery JS, Price DK, and Figg WD (2001). The androgen receptor gene and its influence on the development and progression of prostate cancer. *J Pathol*, **195**, 138–46.

Weigel, NL, and Zhang, Y (1998). Ligand-independent activation of steroid hormone receptors. *J Mol Med*, **76**, 469–79.

Chapter 2

PSA as a marker of progression and response in advanced prostate cancer

Yohann Loriot, Marine Gross-Goupil, and Karim Fizazi

Key points

- Serum PSA is commonly used in prostate cancer patients to assess response to definitive local therapy and to detect relapse after definitive treatment in localized disease
- A low PSA nadir is associated with longer survival after endocrine treatment of metastatic prostate cancer, though survival predictions from PSA parameters are not accurate
- Though PSA is used to evaluate response to chemotherapy and in clinical trials assessing new drugs in prostate cancer, it is unclear whether decline in serum PSA is a surrogate for overall survival
- Physicians should be aware of the postchemotherapy PSA surge syndrome during the first weeks following chemotherapy for CRPC, to preclude early discontinuation of chemotherapy in the erroneous assumption that progression has occurred.

2.1 Introduction

Prostate-specific antigen (PSA) is a 34 kD glycoprotein with protease activity that is found almost exclusively in normal and neoplastic prostate cells and seminal fluid. The production of PSA is mediated by the androgen receptor binding to the androgen response elements in the promoter region of the PSA gene. Serum PSA is commonly used in prostate cancer patients to assess response to definitive local therapy, including radical prostatectomy or radiotherapy , and to detect relapse after definitive treatment in localized disease. The initial PSA value and PSA velocity before treatment have an independent prognostic value in patients with localized disease. Moreover, a dramatic drop in serum PSA measured 3 months after initiating treatment independently correlates with metastasis-free survival in patients treated with androgen deprivation therapy and radiotherapy for high-risk localized disease. Finally, a rapid PSA doubling time and a short interval from radical prostatectomy to the first detectable PSA level are strong and independent prognostic factors in patients with a rising PSA level after local treatment.

PSA is currently used to evaluate response to chemotherapy in patients with castration-resistant prostate cancer (CRPC) and as a marker of response in clinical trials assessing new drugs in prostate cancer. Whether a decline in serum PSA is a surrogate for overall survival or not in metastatic prostate cancer is still debatable. In this regard, the identification of surrogate endpoints capable of replacing true outcome endpoints is crucial to the rapid evaluation of new cancer drugs.

2.2 **PSA and response to endocrine therapy in patients with advanced prostate cancer**

A study reported in 1998 of combined androgen blockade (see reading list) randomly assigned patients who had never received androgen deprivation therapy (ADT) and who had distant metastases from prostate cancer to treatment with bilateral orchiectomy and either flutamide or placebo. There was no significant difference between the two groups in overall survival (p=0.14). The proportion of patients in the flutamide group with at least one PSA measurement of 4.0 ng per milliliter or lower was 74% (95% confidence interval, 69.4 to 78.2), as compared with 61% (95% confidence interval, 56.4 to 66.4) for patients in the placebo group (p<0.001). Thus, the percentage of PSA responses was significantly higher among patients receiving flutamide than among patients receiving the placebo, but patients in the flutamide group did not benefit from significantly better survival. More recently, the Southwest Oncology Group evaluated whether the absolute PSA value after androgen deprivation was prognostic in metastatic prostate cancer. Patients with metastases whose baseline PSA was at least 5 ng/mL underwent induction ADT over 7 months. Patients achieving a PSA level of 4.0 ng/mL or less at months 6 and 7 were randomly assigned to continuous *versus* intermittent ADT at month 8. Eligibility for this analysis required a pre-study PSA determination with at least two subsequent PSA measurements and that patients be registered at least 1 year before the date of the analysis. A PSA level of 4 ng/mL or less after 7 months of ADT was a strong predictor of survival (P < .001).

The EORTC (European Organisation for Research and Treatment of Cancer) studied individual data from 2,161 patients with advanced prostate cancer treated in trials comparing various endocrine therapies using a meta-analytic approach to evaluate whether PSA endpoints could be used as surrogates for overall survival. The patients were randomized between bicalutamide monotherapy and castration or between combined androgen blockade with bicalutamide or flutamide. PSA response, PSA normalization, time to PSA progression, and longitudinal PSA measurements were not strongly correlated with overall survival. The levels of association observed in this study indicate that the effect of hormonal treatment on overall survival cannot be predicted with a high degree of accuracy from the effects of treatment observed on PSA endpoints. Although a correlation between PSA and overall survival was confirmed, the association between the effect of treatment on any PSA endpoint and on overall survival was generally low.

2.3 **PSA, response to chemotherapy, and survival**

Several phase III studies conducted during the 1990's have been analyzed to assess the relationship between the prognosis and PSA variation. An analysis of PSA declines in patients treated with mitoxantrone and prednisone showed that those who achieved a PSA decline of at least 50% had better survival than those who did not, regardless of treatment. Other studies have reported similar data such as the CALGB study comparing mitoxantrone and hydrocortisone to hydrocortisone, and a randomized trial comparing suramin/prednisone to prednisone in men with CRPC. However, these data are of limited significance because there were no statistically significant survival differences between treatment arms.

Two large phase III clinical trials have reported the favorable effect on survival of first-line docetaxel-based chemotherapy in patients with CRPC. A subsequent analysis of the TAX 327 trial explored whether PSA response may be a surrogate endpoint for overall survival. PSA response was defined as a PSA decrease of at least 50% from baseline and confirmed at least 3 weeks later. Only patients with a baseline PSA value of at least 20 ng/mL were evaluated for PSA response. Among the 873 patients evaluable for PSA response, PSA response rates were significantly higher with 3 weekly docetaxel and weekly docetaxel compared with mitoxantrone (45% and 48% versus 32%, respectively; p<0.001 for both). Overall survival was improved in patients evaluable for PSA response receiving 3 weekly docetaxel, with a 25% reduction in the risk of death compared with mitoxantrone (HR, 0.75; 95% CI, 0.61 to 0.94; log rank, p=0.01). Although the weekly docetaxel arm had the highest PSA response rate, it was not associated with increased overall survival compared with mitoxantrone. These data suggest that the beneficial effect of treatment on overall survival in the TAX 327 study is only partially explained by the PSA response.

The second pivotal study (SWOG 99-16) demonstrating an improved survival with docetaxel-estramustine in patients with CRPC has also retrospectively assessed PSA changes as potential surrogate markers for survival. In this trial, men with CRPC were randomly assigned to receive either docetaxel/estramustine (D/E) or mitoxantrone/prednisone (M/P) every three weeks. The results demonstrated a 20% improvement in survival in patients treated with D/E compared with patients treated with M/P. Of 674 eligible patients, 551 had a baseline PSA measurement and at least one PSA measurement during the first 3 months on study. PSA level declines of 5%–90% and PSA velocity at 1, 2, and 3 months were tested for surrogacy for overall survival. Three-month PSA level declines of 20%–40%, a 2-month PSA decline of 30%, and PSA velocity at 2 and 3 months met all three surrogacy criteria whereas PSA level declines of 50% did not meet surrogacy criteria. The optimal biochemical surrogate found in this study was a 30% PSA decline 3 months after treatment initiation. The authors concluded that PSA velocity measured during the first three months after treatment initiation should be taken into account for mortality in further studies in patients with CRPC.

A meta-analytic study assessed PSA response (defined as a decline of 50% or more from baseline level) and PSA progression (defined as a greater than 50% increase above the nadir value) in CRPC patients treated with liarozole, cyproterone acetate or flutamide. This study showed that neither PSA response nor time to PSA progression predicted overall survival. One of the reasons may be that the patients included in this study had very advanced disease and consequently the PSA level might have been affected by any neuroendocrine component of the disease as previously described in this situation.

Other groups have attempted to develop new measures of PSA to define a stronger surrogate for survival. Using a pharmacokinetic principle, a study including 220 CRPC patients treated with docetaxel or mitoxantrone-based chemotherapy aimed to evaluate a new potential predictive factor: the Corrected Area Under the Serum PSA Curve (c-AUC). A retrospective analysis was performed to validate the PSA c-AUC concept, defined as the total Area Under the serum PSA Curve (PSA AUC) value per unit of time, over known PSA values. An abstract of the analysis reported significant difference in overall survival in favor of the low PSA c-AUC level (< 60 ng/mL) group compared with the high PSA c-AUC level (≥ 60 ng/mL) group was observed. The PSA c-AUC variable was the only significant factor in the multivariate analysis. In this regard, in a large retrospective study, PSA kinetics seemed to provide better prediction of survival in metastatic CRPC than all other PSA kinetic variables such as the PSA level halving time after the start of treatment, the PSA level at nadir, the interval to nadir, PSA velocity, and PSA doubling time after reaching the nadir. No prospective data have yet confirmed this study.

Hence, the question of PSA response as a predictive marker of survival remains incompletely answered and requires further prospective evaluation, although a 30% PSA drop was shown to qualify as a surrogate for survival in one study.

2.4 The PSA surge syndrome in patients receiving chemotherapy

A recent study pointed out a new phenomenon, the so-called 'post-chemotherapy PSA surge syndrome' consisting of an initial rise in serum PSA in a high proportion of responders to chemotherapy. This retrospective study included a total of 79 patients with CRPC who received first-line ($n = 52$) or second-line ($n = 27$) chemotherapy. Chemotherapy regimens consisted mainly of docetaxel (with or without estramustine), mitoxantrone-prednisone, doxorubicin-estramustine and irofulven. Among patients who achieved either a response or stabilization, 8 of 41 (20%) had a serum PSA rise during the first 8 weeks of chemotherapy, followed by a subsequent decline in serum PSA. This phenomenon was observed whatever the line of chemotherapy. The postchemotherapy increase in serum PSA in certain cases attained more than twice the baseline value and the duration of the PSA surge ranged from 1 to 8 weeks. No apparent association between the baseline value and the likelihood of observing a surge was reported. Of note, the median progression-free survival duration after the initiation of chemotherapy was 6 months and 3.7 months in patients with an initial PSA surge followed by a PSA response or stabilization, and in those with a response or stabilization but no PSA surge respectively, suggesting that the postchemotherapy PSA surge phenomenon did not negatively impact progression-free survival. Since then, other groups have confirmed these data. In prostate cancer, such a serum PSA rise followed by a PSA drop was previously reported to be a very common occurrence in patients with CRPC receiving consolidation docetaxel-samarium after a response or stabilization following induction chemotherapy. A PSA rise (without cancer progression) during the first year following brachytherapy is also a well-identified feature in patients with localized prostate cancer and is interpreted as PSA secretion due to local inflammation. Moreover, a PSA rise during the first weeks following cryosurgery followed by a subsequent decline has also been reported. It may be hypothesized that this phenomenon corresponds to increased cancer cell destruction, but there is no firm evidence to support this postulate. An alternative hypothesis may include increased differentiation of prostate cancer stem/precursors or enhanced PSA transcriptional efficiency induced by chemotherapy. Physicians should be aware of this postchemotherapy PSA surge syndrome during the first weeks following chemotherapy for CRPC, to preclude early discontinuation of chemotherapy in the erroneous assumption that progression has occurred. As patients are usually aware of their PSA results, they should also be informed of this frequent phenomenon to avoid any undue stress if ever it occurs.

2.5 Conclusion

PSA decline during endocrine therapy or chemotherapy usually indicates a favorable outcome. However, the Prostate Cancer Clinical Trials Working Group recently 'advised against reporting PSA response rates because these are of little value given the uncertain significance of a defined degree of decline from baseline, be it 50% or 30%, and no criterion has been shown prospectively to be a surrogate for clinical benefit' and discouraged the use of changes in PSA-DT or PSA slope as a primary endpoint, because 'their clinical significance is uncertain'. Hence, it recommended that PSA measurements obtained during the first 12 weeks not be used as the sole criterion for clinical decision-making. Physicians and patients should also be aware of the post-chemotherapy surge syndrome to preclude early discontinuation of chemotherapy after inadequate evaluation.

Acknowledgement

The authors thank Lorna de Saint-Ange for editing.

Further reading

Collette L, Burzykowski T, Carroll KJ, Newling D, Morris T, Schröder FH; European Organisation for Research and Treatment of Cancer; Limburgs Universitair Centrum; AstraZeneca Pharmaceuticals (2005). Is prostate-specific antigen a valid surrogate end point for survival in hormonally treated patients with metastatic prostate cancer? Joint research of the European Organisation for Research and Treatment of Cancer, the Limburgs Universitair Centrum, and AstraZeneca Pharmaceuticals. *J Clin Oncol*, **23**, 6139–48.

Dowling AJ, Czaykowski PM, Krahn MD, Moore MJ, Tannock IF (2000). Prostate specific antigen response to mitoxantrone and prednisone in patients with refractory prostate cancer: prognostic factors and generalizability of a multicenter trial to clinical practice. *J Urol*, **163**, 1481–5.

Eisenberger MA, Blumenstein BA, Crawford ED, Miller G, McLeod DG, Loehrer PJ, Wilding G, Sears K, Culkin DJ, Thompson IM Jr, Bueschen AJ, Lowe BA (1998). Bilateral orchiectomy with or without flutamide for metastatic prostate cancer. *N Engl J Med*, **339**, 1036–42.

Hussain M, Tangen CM, Higano C, Schelhammer PF, Faulkner J, Crawford ED, Wilding G, Akdas A, Small EJ, Donnelly B, MacVicar G, Raghavan D; Southwest Oncology Group Trial 9346 (INT-0162) (2006). Absolute prostate-specific antigen value after androgen deprivation is a strong independent predictor of survival in new metastatic prostate cancer: data from Southwest Oncology Group Trial 9346 (INT-0162). *J Clin Oncol*, **24**, 3984–90.

Petrylak DP, Ankerst DP, Jiang CS, Tangen CM, Hussain MH, Lara PN Jr, Jones JA, Taplin ME, Burch PA, Kohli M, Benson MC, Small EJ, Raghavan D, Crawford ED (2006). Evaluation of prostate-specific antigen declines for surrogacy in patients treated on SWOG 99-16. *J Natl Cancer Inst*, **98**, 516–21.

Roessner M, De Wit R, Tannock IF, Yateman N, Yao S, Yver A, Eisenberger MA, on behalf of the TAX 327 Investigators (2005). Prostate-specific antigen (PSA) response as a surrogate endpoint for overall survival (OS): analysis of the TAX327 study comparing docetaxel plus prednisone with mitoxantrone plus prednisone in advanced prostate cancer. *Proc Am Soc Clin Oncol*, **23**, 391s (Abstr 4554).

Robinson D, Sandblom G, Johansson R, Garmo H, Aus G, Hedlund PO, Varenhorst E; Scandinavian Prostate Cancer Group (2008). PSA kinetics provide improved prediction of survival in metastatic hormone-refractory prostate cancer. *Urology*, **72**, 903–7.

Scher HI, Halabi S, Tannock I *et al*; Prostate Cancer Clinical Trials Working Group (2008). Design and End Points of Clinical Trials for Patients With Progressive Prostate Cancer and Castrate Levels of Testosterone: Recommendations of the Prostate Cancer Clinical Trials Working Group. *J Clin Oncol*, **26**, 1148–59.

Small EJ, McMillan A, Meyer M, Chen L, Slichenmyer WJ, Lenehan PF, Eisenberger M (2001). Serum prostate-specific antigen decline as a marker of clinical outcome in hormone-refractory prostate cancer patients: association with progression-free survival, pain end points, and survival. *J Clin Oncol*, **19**, 1304–11.

Smith DC, Dunn RL, Strawderman MS, Pienta KJ (1998). Change in serum prostate-specific antigen as a marker of response to cytotoxic therapy for hormone-refractory prostate cancer. *J Clin Oncol*, **16**, 1835–43.

Thuret R, Massard C, Gross-Goupil M, Escudier B, Di Palma M, Bossi A, de Crevoisier R, Chauchereau A, Fizazi K (2008). The postchemotherapy PSA surge syndrome. *Ann Oncol*, **19**, 1308–11.

Chapter 3

Neo-adjuvant and adjuvant hormone therapy for high-risk localized prostate cancer

Mike D Shelley and Malcolm D Mason

Key points

- Neo-adjuvant or adjuvant hormone therapy enhances the effectiveness of radiotherapy and significantly improves outcomes, including overall survival
- Neo-adjuvant hormone therapy, prior to radical prostatectomy improves pathological variables but not important clinical outcomes
- The role of adjuvant hormone therapy following radical prostatectomy in high risk patients has not yet been established.

3.1 Introduction

The growth of prostate cancer is very sensitive to circulating and prostatic levels of androgens. In prostate tissue, testosterone is converted to 5α-dihydrotestosterone which binds to androgen receptors, leading to growth stimulation. Hormone therapy, more properly referred to as 'Androgen Deprivation Therapy' has been routinely used clinically for decades in the treatment of prostate cancer. Androgen deprivation therapy is the first line of treatment for men with metastatic disease, but here we will consider its role in the management of localized disease. For men whose tumour is confined to the prostate gland, the two major modalitites of treatment are surgery (by radical prostatectomy) or radiotherapy (by extrenal beam therapy, or by brachytherapy). Androgen deprivation therapy may be given before (neo-adjuvant) or after (adjuvant) either of these primary therapies. The aim of neo-adjuvant hormone therapy is to reduce the tumour size and enhance the effectiveness of radiotherapy and facilitate tumour excision during prostatectomy and thus improve patient outcome. Following primary treatment, adjuvant hormone therapy aims to eradicate any residual primary tumour or micro-metastatic disease.

This chapter will overview randomized trials evaluating the effectiveness of adjuvant and neo-adjuvant hormone therapy in patients with high risk localized prostate cancer. Although there is no universal definition of high risk, it is generally defined as those men with any of the following characteristics: Gleason scores >7, a pre-treatment prostate specific antigen (PSA) of > 20ng/ml or clinical stage ≥T3 disease.

3.2 **Hormone therapy combined with radiotherapy**

A number of randomized trials have demonstrated a significantly improved patient outcome when hormone therapy is combined with radiotherapy (Table 3.1). Varying doses and schedules of hormone therapy have been used after radiotherapy and the optimum has yet to be established.

The EORTC 22863 study was a pivotal randomized trial, which administered concurrent and adjuvant hormones to patients with high risk, localized disease, for a period of 3 years, starting on the first day of radiotherapy. This study reported a significant improvement in 5-year overall survival (78% versus 62%, p = 0.0002) and disease-specific survival advantage (94% versus 79%, p = 0.0001) for the combined therapy arm. Clinical disease-free survival was 74% in the combined treatment group which was significantly better than the 40% in the radiotherapy only group (p = 0.0001). A significant improvement was also reported for loco-regional failure (16.4% versus 1.7%, p <0.0001) and in the incidence of distant metastasis (29.2% versus 9.8%, p <0.0001), in favour of adjuvant hormone therapy plus radiotherapy. Treatment related deaths were reported in 1% of patients and grade 3 or 4 late complications were seen in less than 5% of patients. This trial supports the clinical use of adjuvant hormone therapy in node-negative disease.

Table 3.1 Characteristics of randomized studies combining hormone therapy with radical radiotherapy (RT)

Trial	Participants	Interventions	Results
RTOG 8531	Tumour extending beyond prostate (clinical stage T3) or T1 –T2 with regional lymphatic involvement. n = 977	RT alone (prostate dose 70 Gy, pelvic dose 44–46 Gy, 33 fractions) versus RT plus adjuvant Goserelin (3.6 mg s.c. started during last week of treatment and continued indefinitely or until progression).	Adjuvant HT significantly improved rates for overall survival, local failure, distant metastases and disease-specific mortality.
EORTC 22893	412 newly diagnosed T1–2 prostatic cancer of WHO histological grade 3 or T3–4 N0–1 M0 of any histological grade. PSA <20ng/ml in 17% of patients. Gleason score < 7 21%, ≥ 7 33%.	RT alone (50 Gy to pelvis over 5 weeks plus 20 Gy as prostate boost over 2 weeks) versus RT plus adjuvant Goserelin 3.6 mg sc every 4 weeks on 1st day of irradiation for 3 years.	Overall survival, disease-specific survival, disease-free survival, loco-regional failure and the incidence of metastasis were significantly improved with adjuvant HT.
EPCP	1370 T1b-4 M0 Localized disease: T1–2, N0 or Nx, M0. Locally advanced: T3–4 any N, M0 or any T, N+, M0	RT plus placebo versus RT plus adjuvant bicalutamide 150mg/day orally. Median duration of treatment 1.6 years.	Significant improvement in overall survival and progression-free survival, and non-significant improvement in cancer-specific survival for locally advanced disease.
EORTC 22961	970 T1c-2b N1–2 or pN1–2 or T2c-4 N0–2 M0. PSA < 150ng/ml	RT (70Gy) plus 6 months of LHRH agonist versus RT plus 3 years LHRH	No overall survival difference. Biochemical control and progression-free survival improved with 3 year regimen.

Table 3.1 (Contd.)			
Trial	Participants	Interventions	Results
RTOG 8610	456 bulky (5 x 5 cm) T2–4 ± N+	RT (prostate 65–70 Gy, PLN 44–46Gy) alone versus RT plus neoadjuvant HT (Goserelin + Flutamide 2 months before RT and concurrent with RT.	No significant difference in overall survival. Neo-adjuvant HT induced significant improvement in rates for disease-specific mortality, distant metastasis, disease-free survival and biochemical failure.
RTOG 9202	1554 T2c-4 N0M0. PSA < 150ng/ml	RT (65–70 Gy to prostate + 40–50Gy to PLN) plus short-term HT (Goserelin + Flutamide 2 months before and 2 months during RT) versus RT plus long-term HT (as above + 24 months goserelin)	Long-term HT induced significant improvement in overall survival (Gleason 8–10 only), cause-specific survival, disease-free survival, and rates for biochemical failure, local progression and distant metastasis.
Dana-Farber	206 men with localized, T1-T2b, plus one of: PSA > 10, Gleason ≥ 7, extracapsular extension and/or seminal vesicle involvement on endorectal MRI.	RT alone vs RT plus 6 months of maximal androgen blockade.	Increased overall survival in men treated with RT plus hormones, but only in those with no significant comorbidities.

RT=radiotherapy; HT=hormone therapy; PSA=prostatic specific antigen; PLN=pelvic lymph nodes; LHRH=Leutenizing Hormone Releasing Hormone

The RTOG 85-31 trial randomized high-risk patients (predominantly T3 or node positive disease) to radiotherapy alone or radiotherapy plus long-term adjuvant hormone therapy (started in the last week of radiotherapy), and reported the 10-year absolute survival rates as 39% for those not receiving adjuvant therapy and 49% for the adjuvant hormone arm (p = 0.002). Local failure rates were also in favour of adjuvant therapy (23% versus 36%, p <0.001). With a median follow up of 7.6 years for all patients, a significant improvement was shown for disease-specific mortality in the adjuvant treatment group compared to radiotherapy alone (16% and 22%, respectively p < 0.0052). In addition, the incidence of distant metastases in this study was significantly lower for the adjuvant treatment group (p = 0.001). The study showed that adjuvant hormone therapy improves outcomes compared with radiotherapy alone in this group of patients.

One of the largest randomized studies of adjuvant hormone therapy is the Early Prostate Cancer Programme (EPCP), which recruited over 8,000 patients. This programme combined three prospective randomized, placebo-controlled trials of adjuvant bicalutamide, a non-steroidal anti-androgen, in patients receiving radical radiotherapy, radical prostatectomy or watchful waiting. After a median follow up of 7.4 years, the use of adjuvant bicalutamide in those patients receiving radiotherapy, resulted in a significant improvement in overall survival for locally advanced patients (HR 0.65, 95% CI, 1.13–1.84, p = 0.03), but not for the overall population undergoing radiotherapy. The EPCP study reported that there were fewer cancer-related deaths in those patients receiving bicalutamide (16.1% versus 24.3%) compared to radiotherapy alone, although this was only evident in patients with locally advanced disease. There was also a statistically significant improvement in progression-free survival for the bicalutamide group for patients with locally advanced disease (HR 0.58, 95% CI, 0.41 - 0.84, p = 0.003).

Although these studies used different hormone regimens, they tend to indicate that adjuvant hormone therapy provides significant clinical benefit in patients with locally advanced disease but may not be appropriate for men with limited local disease. There are also data to suggest that a longer duration of adjuvant hormone therapy may be more beneficial than shorter durations. The EORTC 22961 phase III trial has reported preliminary data comparing 6 months versus 3 years' adjuvant hormone therapy. Although there was no significant difference in the 5 year overall survival rate (85.3% 3 years versus 80.6% 6 months), clinical progression-free survival (81.8% versus 68.9%) and biochemical progression-free survival (78.3% versus 58.9%) were significantly better with the longer hormone treatment. However, even short-course hormone therapy may be better than no hormone therapy. D'Amico and colleagues recently reported the results of a randomized trial in which patients with high risk, localized disease were treated with radiotherapy alone, or radiotherapy plus 6 months of hormone therapy with maximal androgen blockade (the combination of an LHRH agonist with an anti-androgen). A significant improvement in overall survival was noted in patients treated with combined modality therapy (Hazard Ratio 1.8, p = 0.01), though this benefit was confined to patients without moderate or severe co-morbidities.

One of the first randomized studies to assess the clinical value of short-term hormone therapy given neo-adjuvant to radiotherapy was

RTOG 8610, the long-term results of which have recently been published. In this study patients received radiotherapy alone or radiotherapy plus neo-adjuvant and concurrent hormone therapy. Although overall survival at 10 years was better with hormone therapy, the difference did not reach statistical significance (43% versus 34%, p = 0.12). However, rates for disease-specific mortality (23% versus 36%), distant metastasis (35% versus 47%), biochemical failure (65% versus 80%) and disease-free survival (11% versus 3%) were all significantly in favour of neo-adjuvant hormone therapy. The addition of four months of neo-adjuvant hormone therapy with radiotherapy appears to provide substantial clinical benefit in patients with bulky localized or locally advanced prostate cancer, and appears to be well tolerated.

A longer period of hormone therapy also seems to have clinical benefits when administered in the neoadjuvant plus adjuvant setting. The RTOG 9202 randomized trial investigated the optimum duration of hormone therapy. There was no significant difference in the 5 year overall survival rate when hormone therapy was given over 4 months or 28 months (78.5% versus 80.0%, respectively p = 0.73). The 4 month treatment comprised 2 months neoadjuvant and 2 months concomitant ADT. The longer treatment added 24 months of adjuvant ADT. However, a subset analysis indicated a significant overall survival advantage in patients with Gleason scores 8 – 10 receiving the longer duration schedule (81.0% versus 70.7%, p = 0.044). Long-term hormone therapy also showed a significant improvement in all other treatment outcomes at 5 years.

3.3 Hormone therapy combined with radical prostatectomy

The role of hormone therapy combined with radical prostatectomy has been evaluated in many randomized trials although the majority have been centred on neo-adjuvant therapy. Substantial data on adjuvant therapy are limited to a few large randomized studies (Table 3.2).

An oft-cited study is the ECOG EST 3886 trial which evaluated the timing of adjuvant hormone therapy after radical prostatectomy and pelvic lymphadenectomy in men with node positive prostate cancer. Patients were recruited from 36 USA centres and randomly assigned to immediate or delayed hormone therapy, the latter administered on evidence of disease recurrence or metastasis. At a median follow up of 11.9 years overall survival was significantly better in the immediate hormonal treatment arm compared to the control arm (HR 1.84, 95% confidence interval 1.01–3.35; p = 0.04). There was also a

Table 3.2 Characteristics of randomized studies combining adjuvant hormone therapy with prostatectomy

Trial	Participants	Interventions	Results
ECOG EST 3886	Men who had undergone radical prostatectomy and bilateral pelvic lymphadenectomy for clinically localized disease (stage T2 or less with nodal metastases). Median age 65.6 y (range: 45–78 y) Detectable PSA 20%, elevated acid phosphatase 12%. Gleason score <7 65%, ≥7 35% (median 7).	RP alone with delayed hormone therapy (n = 40) versus RP plus immediate hormone therapy (either goserelin 3.6 mg sc every 28 days until progression or bilateral orchidectomy, n = 38).	Immediate hormone therapy significantly improved overall survival, cancer-specific survival and progression-free survival compared to delayed therapy.
German Multicentre Trial	Men with pT3–4pN0 prostate cancer, any PSA level and grade (median 64, range 41–78). Tumour grades were G1 9%, G2 55%, G3 36%.	RP alone (n = 157) versus RP plus adjuvant flutamide 250 mg orally three times a day (total 750 mg a day) indefinitely (n = 152).	Minimal difference in overall survival. Recurrence-free survival significantly better with adjuvant hormone therapy.
	T1-4 M0 any N prostate cancer clinically or pathologically confirmed. (mean age 67 years).	RP plus placebo versus RP plus adjuvant bicalutamide (150 mg orally once a day). Numbers randomized unclear.	No significant difference in overall survival. Adjuvant bicalutamide significantly improved progression-free survival.

RP=radical prostatectomy; PSA=prostate-specific antigen.

statistically significant improvement in disease-specific survival (HR 4.09, 95% confidence interval 1.76–9.49; p = 0.0004) and progression-free survival (HR 3.42, 95% confidence interval 1.96-5.98; p < 0.0001) in favour of immediate adjuvant hormone therapy. In this study serum PSA was not used as a marker for eligibility or disease recurrence as recruitment began before the usefulness of this marker was fully recognized. In addition, in current clinical practice with careful patient selection, relatively few patients undergoing radical prostatectomy are subsequently found to have microscopic nodal metastases, and the relevance of this trial to contemporary practice should be viewed with caution.

A German multi-centre, prospective randomized trial has reported on adjuvant hormone therapy versus observation in men with node negative disease. In contrast to the ECOG EST 3886 trial, this German study, at a median follow up of 6.1 years, showed little difference in overall survival between study groups (HR 1.04, 95% confidence interval 0.53–2.02; p = 0.92). However, a significant improvement in recurrence-free survival was observed in men receiving the adjuvant therapy (p = 0.0041 log rank). It was noted that toxicity was considerably more common in the adjuvant arm (43% versus 3%) and discontinuation of treatment was twice that of the control group.

The Early Prostate Cancer Programme (EPCP) evaluating adjuvant bicalutamide included 4454 patients who underwent radical prostatectomy. Tolerability and efficacy of adjuvant oral bicalutamide were assessed. With long-term follow up this study reported no improvement in overall survival with bicalutamide in either the local (HR 1.0, 95% CI, 0.80–1.26) or the locally advanced (HR 1.09, 95% CI, 0.85–1.39, p = 0.51) subgroups. However, there was a significant improvement in progression-free survival after a median of 7.4 years (HR 0.75, 95% CI, 0.61–0.91, p = 0.004). This result was for a combined group of local and locally advanced patients and was highly influenced by the much better response observed in patients with locally advanced disease. The major side-effects of adjuvant bicalutamide were breast pain (73%) and gynaecomastia (69%) which were mild to moderate in about 90% of cases. Twenty-nine percent of patients withdrew from active treatment due to adverse events compared to 10% for the control groups. The data from this study suggest that bicalutamide adjuvant to prostatectomy has little benefit for men with early localized disease but may have some clinical advantage with locally advanced disease.

There have been several randomized studies of neo-adjuvant hormones prior to prostatectomy over the last 10 to 15 years. These have varied in the type of hormonal therapy administered, some using single agents, either an anti-androgen or LHRH analogue, whilst others have used combined androgen blockade. Patients have been predominantly those with T1 and T2 disease. All the studies to date have shown that neo-adjuvant hormones prior to radical prostatectomy substantially improve local pathological variables although the optimum schedule has not been determined. The positive surgical margin rate is significantly lower in patients receiving hormone therapy compared to those having radical prostatectomy alone. In addition, the rates for organ confinement and positive lymph node involvement are significantly improved with neo-adjuvant hormone therapy, although the rate for seminal vesicle invasion appears to be unaffected. Longer durations of adjuvant therapy appear to enhance these positive pathological effects. However, the improvement in pathological factors with neo-adjuvant hormone therapy did not translate to a similar benefit in terms of overall survival. No study has shown a difference in overall survival or disease-specific survival in patients receiving neo-adjuvant hormone therapy. Therefore the value of neo-adjuvant hormone before prostatectomy is not convincing and is generally not recommended outside clinical trials.

3.4 **Discussion**

Improving survival rates over the last few decades for men with prostate cancer illustrate that significant advances have been made in the management of this disease. However, a considerable number of men develop progressive disease following radiotherapy or prostatectomy and are not cured. There is, therefore, an urgent need to enhance the effectiveness of existing therapies and improve the outlook of men who are at high risk of failure. Evaluating the role of hormone therapy in combination with radiotherapy or prostatectomy has resulted in some encouraging data.

The results from randomized trials clearly demonstrate that adjuvant, neoadjuvant, or concurrent hormone therapy may improve outcomes in patients undergoing radiotherapy. The absence of overlapping toxicities makes this combination an attractive approach.

It is known from *in vitro* data that both hormone therapy and radiotherapy induce tumour cell killing by apoptosis, but probably by different mechanisms. This differential effect could result in the eradication of both hormone sensitive and hormone independent tumour cells. This may account for the additive or synergistic of hormone therapy when combined with radiotherapy. Alternatively, the systemic effect of hormone therapy on occult micro-metastases might account for some of its therapeutic effect.

Although hormone therapy combined with radiotherapy is an active therapeutic option for men with high risk prostate cancer, it is associated with significant side-effects. Most recently, attention has focused on the risks of cardiovascular disease, consequent upon the development of a metabolic syndrome, in patients undergoing hormone therapy. Therefore, for men considering this therapeutic option, their decision should be an informed one based on its efficacy and risks. The role of hormone therapy with brachytherapy remains to be established.

Although hormone therapy neo-adjuvant to radical prostatectomy has a positive effect on surgical margin status, it is not clear whether this is due to tumour cell death or difficulties in pathological interpretation because of cellular architectural changes induced by hormone therapy. Although tumour volume may be reduced with neo-adjuvant hormones therapy, there does not seem to be a concomitant improvement in the surgical procedure in terms of operation time and blood loss. Taking these factors into account and the lack of a significant clinical benefit, hormone therapy neo-adjuvant to prostatectomy should not be routinely offered to men with high-risk prostate cancer.

There are limited data from randomized trials on the efficacy of hormone therapy adjuvant to radical prostatectomy and the issue remains controversial. There is no clear indication that overall survival is improved although disease progression may be delayed. However, some of these data are immature and because of the protracted nature of prostate cancer, longer follow up may be required to determine the true effect of this treatment option.

Even after decades of clinical use, there remain unresolved issues with regard to the optimization of hormone therapy used in combination with radiotherapy. Questions remain concerning the choice of hormonal agent, and what dose and schedule should be employed. There is a case for individual tailoring of hormone therapy for each patient depending on their volume of disease and other risk parameters.

Further reading

D'Amico A, Chen M-H, Renshaw AA, Loffredo M, Kantoff PW (2008). Androgen suppression and radiation vs radiation alone for prostate cancer. A randomized trial. *JAMA*, **299**, 289–95.

Bolla M, Collette L, Blank L, Warde P, Dubois JB, Mirimanoff R-O, Storme G, Bernier J, Kuten A, Sternberg C, Mattelaer J, Torecilla JL, Pfeffer JR, Cutajar CL, Zurio A, Pierart M (2002). Long-term results with immediate androgen suppression and external irradiation in patients with locally advanced prostate cancer (an EORTC study): a Phase III randomised trial. *The Lancet*, **360**, 193–208.

Hanks G, Pajak TF, Porter A, Grignon D, Brereton H, Venkatesan V, Horwitz EM, Lawton C, Tosenthal SA, Sandler HM, Shipley WU (2003). Phase III trial of long-term adjuvant androgen deprivation after neoadjuvant hormonal cytoreduction and radiotherapy in locally advanced carcinoma of the prostate: The Radiation Therapy Oncology Group Protocol 92-02. *J Clin Oncol*, **21**(21), 3872–978.

Messing EM, Manola J, Yao G, Kiernan M, Crawford D, Wilding G, di'SantAgnes PA, Trump D, on behalf of the Eastern Cooperative Oncology Group study EST 3886 (2006). Immediate versus delayed androgen deprivation treatment in patients with node-positive prostate cancer after radical prostatectomy and pelvic lymphadenectomy. *Lancet Oncol*, **7**, 472–9.

Pilepich MV, Winter K, Lawton C, Krish RF, Wolkov HB, Movsas B, Hug EB, Asbell SO, Grignon D (2005). Androgen suppression adjuvant to definitive radiotherapy in prostate carcinoma—long-term results of phase III RTOG 85-31 (2005). *Int J Radiat Oncol Biol Phys*, **61** (5), 1285–90.

Roach M, Bae K, Speight J, Wolkov HB, Rubin P, Lee RJ, Lawton C, Valicenti R, Grignon D, Pilepich MV (2008). Short-term neoadjuvant androgen deprivation therapy and external-beam radiotherapy for locally advanced prostate cancer: Long-term results of RTOG 8610. *J Clin Oncol*, **26**(4), 585–91.

Tyrrell C, Payne H, See WA, McLeod DG, Wirth MP, Iversen P, Armstrong J, Morris C, on behalf of the 'Casodex' Early Prostate Cancer Trialists' Group. Bicalutamide ('Casodex') 150mg as adjuvant to radiotherapy in patients with localised or locally advanced prostate cancer: Results from the randomised Early Prostate Cancer Programme (2005). *Radiother Oncol*, **76**, 4–10.

Wirth MP, Weissbach L, Marx F-J, Heckl W, Jellinghaus W, Reidmiller H, Noack B, Hinke A, Froechner M (2004). Prospective randomised trial comparing Flutamide as adjuvant treatment versus observation after radical prostatectomy for locally advanced lymph node negative prostate cancer. *Eur Urol*, **45**, 267–70.

Chapter 4

Systemic treatment of recurrence after local therapies

Daniel M Moreira, Stephen J Freedland,
Judd W Moul, and Lionel L Bañez

Key points

- Biochemical recurrence (BCR) is defined as prostate-specific antigen (PSA) rise above 0.2ng/mL after radical prostatectomy and PSA value greater than nadir plus 2ng/mL after other local therapies
- Patients with local recurrence after local therapies may benefit from local salvage therapies (e.g. salvage prostatectomy or salvage radiotherapy)
- Surgical castration and luteinizing hormone-releasing hormone (LHRH) agonists are currently first-line systemic therapy for prostate cancer recurrence after local therapies
- Hormonal therapy is associated with sexual dysfunction, cognitive impairment, osteoporosis, lipid abnormalities, loss of muscle mass, anemia, diabetes, and cardiovascular disease
- Androgen deprivation therapy (ADT) for PSA-only relapse should be reserved for patients with high risk of progression wherein benefits of ADT outweighs risks for its side-effects.

4.1 Recurrence after local therapies

Approximately 80–90% of patients diagnosed with prostate cancer in the USA will undergo definitive local therapy and about 30–35% will develop disease recurrence. Initially, the majority of these patients are asymptomatic and PSA elevation is the only indication of disease relapse. The natural history after failure of local therapies is usually slowly progressive but can be quite variable. Pound *et al.* demonstrated that in absence of early hormonal therapy the median time to develop clinically-evident metastasis was 8 years from time of PSA elevation and 5 years from metastasis to death. In a follow-up study, the median time from PSA recurrence to prostate cancer death was not reached after 16 years' post-treatment.

4.1.1 Recurrence after radical prostatectomy

Approximately 25–45% of patients diagnosed with prostate cancer will undergo radical prostatectomy. Even though the recurrence-free survival after surgery has been increasing, about 15–40% of patients will develop recurrence within 5 years. BCR after radical prostatectomy is defined as a PSA rise above 0.2ng/mL or two consecutive PSA determinations of 0.2ng/mL. Adjuvant radiotherapy can reduce the risk of recurrence in those with adverse features, but may not be a better policy than sensitive PSA monitoring, with radiotherapy on early biochemical failure.

4.1.2 Recurrence after radiotherapy

Approximately 15–30% of patients with diagnosis of prostate cancer will undergo external beam radiotherapy (ERBT) or brachytherapy. About 10% of low-risk and up to 60% of high-risk patients will experience BCR. A recent consensus (Phoenix criteria) defines BCR after radiotherapy as a PSA value greater than absolute nadir plus 2ng/mL, PSA greater than current nadir plus 3ng/mL or 2 consecutive increases of at least 0.5ng/mL.

4.1.3 Recurrence after other local therapies

For other local therapies such as cryoablation and high-intensity focused ultrasound, though no clear standards have been set; BCR is often defined as a PSA value greater than nadir plus 2ng/mL.

4.2 Predicting disease progression

Given that the natural history of PSA recurrence is variable and generally long, it is important to determine which patients will develop disease progression and may eventually die from prostate cancer and which patients will have a long and indolent course and will ultimately die from other causes. Stratification according to risk of disease progression serves to identify patients that may benefit from more aggressive approaches (e.g. early salvage treatment). The most accepted predictors of disease progression are high Gleason score, short PSA doubling time (PSADT) and short time interval between surgery and PSA elevation. Gleason score of 8–10 confers a significant worse prognosis after recurrence. Though the association between short PSADT and risk of prostate cancer death is on a continuum, a PSADT <9 months is particularly an ominous factor for progression. Early BCR, especially within 3 years for surgical patients, is also associated with increased risk of disease progression.

4.3 Treatment options for BCR after local therapies

It is important to determine whether the cause of PSA elevation is local failure only or distant disease recurrence. Local recurrence can potentially be cured by local salvage treatment (e.g. salvage EBRT or salvage prostatectomy). Although there are no tests to accurately differentiate these two clinical situations, factors such as disease-free interval, Gleason score and pathological staging are helpful in determining the risk of systemic recurrence. While imaging tests do exists (e.g. bone scan, MRI, prostascint, PET scan), in general their sensitivity and specificity are less than ideal when PSA is very low and decisions need to be made.

4.3.1 Salvage EBRT

The reported success rates of salvage EBRT after failure following radical prostatectomy range between 10–50%. A recent retrospective study showed that salvage radiotherapy administered within 2 years of BCR in patients with localized prostate cancer after prostatectomy is associated with a significant >80% reduction in risk of prostate cancer-specific mortality in men with PSADT <6 months.

4.3.2 Salvage radical prostatectomy

Historically salvage prostatectomy for men with recurrence after EBRT was rarely performed due to concerns about lack of efficacy and high morbidity. However, two large series found 10-year prostate cancer specific survival rates of 65–73%. In highly selected patients complication rates approach those in men with primary radical prostatectomy and quality of life outcomes are only modestly worse, suggesting for selected men, this may be a reasonable approach.

4.3.3 Androgen deprivation therapy

ADT refers to treatments meant to eliminate testosterone production (surgical or pharmacological castration), prevent testosterone binding to cellular receptors or a combination. It is the most commonly used salvage therapy for prostate cancer. However, unlike local salvage therapies, which are aimed at cure, hormonal therapy is not curative. In metastatic disease, ADT improves symptoms and prolongs survival, thus it is the standard treatment for advanced cases. In BCR, where symptoms are usually absent, it is not clear which patient group will benefit from this treatment and which may actually be harmed by its side-effects. Unfortunately, due to lack of randomized trials of ADT in BCR, several aspects of ADT for PSA-relapse are unknown. Currently, most of the best evidence on ADT for BCR relies on retrospective studies or data extrapolated from patients with advanced disease.

The real benefit of ADT in non-metastatic PSA recurrence remains the subject of much debate. While some studies have suggested that early ADT after PSA elevation may delay metastasis or improve overall survival, these findings are based upon retrospective analysis. Thus, no prospective randomized study has addressed this question. Given this uncertainty, to answer this question, we must extrapolate findings from other disease settings. For example, in men with metastatic or locally advanced disease, early ADT improves prostate cancer survival and has only modest or no affect on overall survival. Moreover, it is known that ADT has significant side-effects including cardiovascular disease, diabetes, and perhaps increased non-prostate cancer mortality. Indeed, in 2006, the American Society of Clinical Oncology (ASCO) updated their guidelines for initial ADT and concluded that 'In metastatic or progressive prostate cancer, immediate versus symptom-onset institution of ADT results in a moderate decrease (17%) in relative risk (RR) for prostate cancer mortality, a moderate increase (15%) in RR for non–prostate cancer-specific mortality, and no overall survival advantage'. Thus, it seems reasonable to use early aggressive ADT for men at the greatest risk of prostate cancer death (e.g. those with short PSADT). Again, while the degree to which this approach reduces prostate cancer mortality is currently unknown, the alternative—to delay hormones until disease progression—is associated with a very high mortality rate, especially for those with a PSADT <9 months. Therefore, given the choice between a treatment with an uncertain benefit and a near certain death, we would advise the treatment with uncertain benefit. Alternatively, those who are at the lowest risk of prostate cancer death (e.g. those with long PSADT) are very unlikely to have disease progression even without further treatment. As such, these men can be relatively safely spared from ADT toxicity.

4.3.3.1 *Surgical castration*

Bilateral orchiectomy quickly reduces circulating testosterone levels and has been proven to reduce pain and increase survival in patients with advanced disease. It is a simple, safe, and inexpensive outpatient procedure that can be performed under local anesthesia. It is considered the 'gold-standard' ADT which other treatments are compared to.

4.3.3.2 *Luteinizing hormone–releasing hormone agonists*

LHRH agonists have become the current standard form of hormonal treatment for prostate cancer. The degree of androgen blockade and profile of side-effects are comparable to those seen in patients subjected to surgical castration. Although agonist, steady elevated levels of LHRH cause inhibition of gonadotropin release. LHRH agonists are commonly used along with anti-androgens at the beginning of treatment to prevent deleterious effects of transiently elevated testosterone. All drugs in this group have similar actions and side-effect profiles. See Table 4.1 for medications and dosages. LHRH agonists and antagonists equivalently suppress testosterone production. The main advantages of antagonists are their fast action and their direct antagonistic activity that eliminates testosterone flare and the need of anti-androgen co-administration. However, they are associated with potential allergic reactions, even after previously uneventful treatment.

Table 4.1 Androgens deprivation therapy regimens

Drug group	Drug name	Routes	Dosages	Dosing interval
LHRH agonist	Goserelin	sc	3.6mg	Every month
			10.8mg	Every 3 months
	Leuprorelin	i.m. or sc	7.5mg[a]	Every month
			22.5mg	Every 3 months
			30mg	Every 4 months
		Implant	65mg	Yearly
	Triptorelin	i.m.	3.75mg	Every month
			11.25mg	Every 3 months
	Histrelin[c]	Implant	50mg	Yearly
LRHR antagonist	Abarelix[c]	i.m.	100mg	Every month
	Degarelix[c]	sc	80mg[b]	Every month
Anti-androgen	Bicalutamide	Oral	50–150mg[d]	Daily
	Flutamide	Oral	250mg	Three times daily
	Nilutamide[c]	Oral	150–300mg	Daily
	Cyproterone*	Oral	100mg	Two-three times daily
Estrogen	Diethylstilbestrol*	Oral	1–3mg	Daily

* Not FDA-approved for use in the United States, but approved in some European countries.
[a] These are USA doses, in Europe the dose is 3.75mg monthly or 11.25mg 3-monthly.
[b] After first month loading dose of 240mg.
[c] Not licensed in the UK.
[d] 150mg dose as a single agent.

4.3.3.3 *Anti-androgens*

Anti-androgens act as competitors of androgens at receptor level. They are further divided in steroidal anti-androgens (cyproterone) and non-steroidal anti-androgens (flutamide, bicalutamide, nilutamide). Non-steroidal anti-androgens are pure anti-androgens and do not suppress testosterone secretion. Steroidal anti-androgens have progestational activity that decreases serum testosterone levels, leading to loss of libido and sexual dysfunction.

There are limited data on efficacy of cyproterone as monotherapy especially for BCR. Nevertheless, it has been used not only as monotherapy but as an agent to prevent disease flare (*see LHRH Agonists*) or in combined androgen blockade (CAB). No studies established an optimal dose; the most common regimen, however, is 100mg three times a day. Based on current data, the only advantage of cyproterone over castration appears to be the lower incidence of hot flushes. In addition, cyproterone use is strongly associated with cardiovascular side-effects and adverse changes in serum lipoproteins and carbohydrate metabolism, and thus its use is not approved by Food and Drug Administration (FDA) and it is not used in the United States.

Flutamide is the oldest drug in the non-steroidal anti-androgen group. Optimal dosage has not been established, but usual regimen is 250mg three times a day. Diarrhoea and liver toxicity are common side-effects. Nilutamide is usually given 150mg daily and it is associated with a higher incidence of adverse effects, particularly interstitial pneumonitis and delayed adaptation to darkness. Bicalutamide, the most widely studied and prescribed drug of this group, is given once a day (50–150mg). It is the most potent and best tolerated among non-steroidal anti-androgens. One study compared high dose bicalutamide (150mg) daily to surgical castration and showed similar survival for locally-advanced non-metastatic disease with similar or slightly better quality of life outcomes. Results from Early Prostate Cancer trial indicate that early or adjuvant anti-androgen therapy with high dose bicalutamide prolongs progression-free survival in patients with locally advanced prostate cancer, irrespective of primary therapy. However, only as adjuvant therapy after EBRT, did early ADT prolong overall survival. In men with low-risk, localized prostate cancer undergoing watchful waiting, 150mg bicalutamide was associated with significantly worse overall survival compared to those on placebo, further underscoring potential toxicity of any form of ADT for those with low-risk disease.

4.3.3.4 *Estrogens*

Oral estrogens are effective in controlling symptoms and decreasing risk of dying from prostate cancer. However, due to a high incidence of cardiovascular side-effects, oral estrogens are not commonly used nowadays, except in extraordinary situations. Estrogens patches are being evaluated in metastatic disease but no studies in biochemical failure are available at present.

4.3.3.5 Other agents

In one small study, finasteride use in association with anti-androgens for PSA relapse after primary treatment was associated with improved PSA control. Hard outcome data such as prevention of metastasis and overall survival, however, is not available. Other ADT agents such as aminoglutethimide, abiraterone, and ketoconazole have not been evaluated in non-metastatic prostate cancer recurrence.

4.3.3.6 Combined androgen blockade

The reason for concomitant use of two or more forms of ADT is based on the idea that after elimination of testicular androgens, adrenal androgens still contribute to prostate cancer progression. The most commonly used combination is LHRH agonist with an anti-androgen. Many studies have addressed its efficacy in metastatic disease with mixed results, providing data to support either opinion. A recent meta-analysis of CAB using non-steroidal anti-androgens in men with metastatic disease suggests a relative 7–20% decrease in prostate cancer death. However, its efficacy in non-metastatic disease remains to be determined.

4.3.3.7 Timing of ADT

Differences between early and delayed salvage ADT for PSA recurrence were examined by two retrospective studies. Moul et al. did not find a significant overall difference in risk of developing metastasis between early and delayed therapy (starting when PSA was lower or greater than 5ng/mL) among men who failed radical prostatectomy. However, in patients at high risk of progression (Gleason score >=8 or PSADT <12 months) early ADT was associated with a 50% decrease in risk of developing metastasis after a median follow-up of 3.7 years. A separate study demonstrated an increase in overall survival in men that received ADT with a PSA <20ng/mL after radiotherapy. Therefore, for high-risk men, early ADT may decrease metastasis and prolong overall and progression-free survival but it is counterbalanced by its side-effects as discussed below.

4.3.3.8 Intermittent ADT

In an attempt to reduce ADT toxicity, there has been increased interest in intermittent ADT. Currently, three phase III trials are underway examining whether intermittent hormonal therapy results in survival rates similar to or better than those of continuous hormonal therapy while preserving better quality of life. However, to date there are no data to support whether intermittent therapy is better or worse than continuous therapy in terms of its effect on survival. Until more mature data are available it is difficult to argue for or against intermittent therapy as a viable therapeutic option.

4.3.3.9 *ADT side-effects*

ADT has been traditionally linked to development of sexual dysfunction, cognitive impairment, osteoporosis, lipid abnormalities, loss of muscle mass and anemia. Nearly all regimens are also associated with hot flushes and gynecomastia. More recently, cardiovascular and metabolic side-effects have been better characterized. ADT was shown to be associated with up to 40% increased risk of diabetes and 10% increased risk of cardiovascular disease in population level analyses. Several studies have now suggested that ADT use is associated with a significant increase in risk of death from cardiovascular causes. These important side-effects should be taken into account when deciding to start ADT.

4.3.4 **Non-hormonal systemic treatments**

A number of substances have been investigated as possible alternative to ADT for rising PSA. COX-2 inhibitors, for example, were shown to slow the rate of PSA rising after local treatments. Similarly, pomegranate juice, in a non-randomized study has been shown to slow PSADT. In hormone resistant disease, new drugs such as sunitinib, atrasentan, and bevacizumab are being tested with mixed results but none of them have been evaluated in PSA-only elevation. Chemotherapy agents such as docetaxel have been shown to improve survival for patients with androgen-independent disease. Currently, three trials are addressing the early use of docetaxel after local therapy and results will be available in the near future.

4.4 **Secondary rising PSA after systemic treatment**

Also known as non-metastatic castration-refractory prostate cancer, this entity has become more common due to use of early ADT. A retrospective study showed a 33% incidence of metastasis within 2 years after secondary PSA rise and a median bone metastasis free survival of 30 months in this group of patients. Unfortunately, no standard treatment is currently available. The use of a secondary ADT (e.g. bicalutamide, estrogens, or ketoconazole) has been studied with mixed results. The most commonly used strategy is to add anti-androgens to the current regimen. In patients already receiving CAB, withdrawal of anti-androgens have been shown to elicit a biochemical response in 15–20%. (See Chapter 6: Second and third-line hormone therapies).

Further reading

Efstathiou, JA, Bae, K, Shipley, WU, Hanks, GE, Pilepich, MV, Sandler, H.M & Smith, MR (2008). Cardiovascular Mortality and Duration of Androgen Deprivation for Locally Advanced Prostate Cancer: Analysis of RTOG 92–02. *Eur Urol*, **54**, 816–23.

Freedland, SJ, Humphreys, EB, Mangold, LA, Eisenberger, M., Dorey, FJ, Walsh, PC & Partin, AW (2005). Risk of prostate cancer-specific mortality following biochemical recurrence after radical prostatectomy. *JAMA*, **294**, 433–9.

Isbarn, H, Boccon-Gibod, L, Carroll, PR, Montorsi, F, Schulman, C, Smith, MR, Sternberg, CN & Studer, UE (2008). Androgen Deprivation Therapy for the Treatment of Prostate Cancer: Consider Both Benefits and Risks. *Eur Urol* Oct 14.

Loblaw, DA, Virgo, KS, Nam, R, Somerfield, MR, Ben-Josef, E, Mendelson, DS, Middleton, R, Sharp, SA, Smith, TJ, Talcott, J, Taplin, M, Vogelzang, NJ, Wade, JL, 3rd, Bennett, CL & Scher, HI (2007). Initial hormonal management of androgen-sensitive metastatic, recurrent, or progressive prostate cancer: 2006 update of an American Society of Clinical Oncology practice guideline. *J Clin Oncol*, **25**, 1596–605.

Moul, JW, Wu, H, Sun, L, Mcleod, DG, Amling, C, Donahue, T, Kusuda, L, Sexton, W, O'reilly, K, Hernandez, J, Chung, A & Soderdahl, D (2004). Early versus delayed hormonal therapy for prostate specific antigen only recurrence of prostate cancer after radical prostatectomy. *J Urol*, **171**, 1141–7.

Pound, CR, Partin, AW, Eisenberger, MA, Chan, DW, Pearson, JD & Walsh, PC (1999). Natural history of progression after PSA elevation following radical prostatectomy. *JAMA*, **281**, 1591–7.

Siddiqui, SA, Boorjian, SA, Inman, B, Bagniewski, S, Bergstralh, EJ & Blute, ML (2008). Timing of androgen deprivation therapy and its impact on survival after radical prostatectomy: a matched cohort study. *J Urol*, **179**, 1830–7.

Wirth, MP, Weissbach, L, Marx, FJ, Heckl, W, Jellinghaus, W, Riedmiller, H, Noack, B, Hinke, A & Froehner, M (2004). Prospective randomized trial comparing flutamide as adjuvant treatment versus observation after radical prostatectomy for locally advanced, lymph node-negative prostate cancer. *Eur Urol*, **45**, 267–70.

Chapter 5

First-line hormonal therapy for metastatic prostate cancer

Ajjai S Alva and Maha Hussain

Key points

- Androgen deprivation therapy ((ADT) gonadal suppression) is the standard first line therapy for patients with metastatic prostate cancer. This can be accomplished medically with the use of an LHRH-agonist or antagonist or by bilateral orchiectomy
- The addition of an anti-androgen (short course or continuous) must be individualized taking into account symptoms, sides effects, and costs of therapy
- Pending results of completed randomized trials, intermittent androgen deprivation therapy can be used but is considered experimental
- Physicians managing patients should attend to the long-term toxicity from ADT, particularly effect on BMD and the metabolic syndromes
- Considering the inevitability of progression in virtually all patients undergoing ADT, new treatment strategies targeting mechanisms of progression are an active area of investigation.

5.1 Introduction

The critical role of androgens in prostate cancer growth and the potential for therapeutic utility in treating it by blocking androgens were described by Huggins and Hodges in 1941. Androgen deprivation therapy (ADT) is now well established as the primary treatment for metastatic prostate cancer and plays a key role as well in the treatment of localized and locally advanced disease.

Despite high subjective and objective response rates nearly all patients with metastatic disease treated with ADT will eventually progress despite castrate levels of testosterone—a clinical state termed castration refractory prostate cancer, over a median of 18–24 months. There are several potential controversies in the use of first line ADT in metastatic prostate cancer. Key questions include when to start treatment, what modalities to use and what schedule. In this chapter, we discuss the current indications for first-line androgen deprivation therapy in metastatic prostate cancer with the available evidence, the unsettled controversies over methods, timing and mode of hormonal blockade, the most commonly used agents in ADT, the monitoring of such therapy and the prognostic markers that may be potentially useful in clinical decision-making.

5.2 **Physiology**

Prostate cancer is an androgen-driven cancer. The hypothalamic-pituitary-gonadal (HPG) axis regulates the synthesis and secretion of androgens from the testes, the major site of androgen production. GnRH (gonadotropin-releasing hormone) is secreted by the hypothalamus and is transported to the anterior pituitary via the hypophyseal portal vein. In the anterior pituitary, GnRH acts on GnRH receptors to stimulate secretion of LH (luteinizing hormone) and FSH (follicle stimulating hormone). GnRH is therefore also known as LHRH (luteinizing hormone-releasing hormone). LH and FSH are secreted into the bloodstream and act on the testes to stimulate testosterone and inhibin secretion respectively. The HPG axis is regulated by negative feedback loops of testosterone and inhibin on the anterior pituitary and/or hypothalamus. Testosterone is converted to dihyrdrotestoserone (DHT) by the enzyme 5-alpha reductase. DHT has much greater affinity for the androgen receptor (AR) in target organs than testosterone itself. AR modulates expression of several downstream genes and pathways in the prostate cell that promote survival and growth.

5.3 **Methods of ADT**

5.3.1 **Primary gonadal suppression**

5.3.1.1 *Surgical castration*

Bilateral orchiectomy is the gold standard method to achieve gonadal testosterone deprivation and an accepted first line hormonal therapy for advanced prostate cancer. Advantages of lower cost, simplicity, and low morbidity of the procedure and rapidity of attaining castrate testosterone levels with resultant relief of pain and other symptoms are however counter-balanced by the considerable psychological impact of the surgery and the lack of reversibility particularly given the younger age at diagnosis in the PSA era. In one questionnaire-based study, only 22% of eligible men opted for surgical castration compared to medical alternatives. Advances such as subcapsular orchiectomy and testicular prostheses have not changed this scenario.

5.3.1.2 *LHRH agonists*

LHRH (GnRH) agonists bind to GnRH receptors in the anterior pituitary, causing an initial transient increase in LH release and rise in testosterone levels. Subsequently, GnRH receptors are down regulated in the second week resulting in a decline in testosterone levels to the castrate range over the next 3–4 weeks. The initial testosterone 'flare' can be avoided particularly in patients with symptoms or impending symptoms by starting a lead-in anti-androgen prior to starting LHRH agonist therapy. It is reasonable to consider 7–10 days of anti-androgens before LHRH and continuing for at least 2 weeks after. This is especially important to avoid worsening pain and precipitating possible spinal cord and ureteral obstruction by critically-located metastatic disease. A recently reported alternative would be the use of an LHRH antagonist such as degarelix, since testosterone flare is avoided. This drug was approved in the US in January 2009.

Administration: LHRH agonists include leuprolide, goserelin and triptorelin. Depot formulations of leuprorelin are commonly used as intramuscular injections every 1 month (7.5 mg), 3 months (22.5 mg) or 4 months (30 mg) though longer acting formulations are available up to 1 year as subcutaneous implants. Goserelin is given as 3.6 mg sc injections every month or 10.8 mg sc injections every 3 months. Triptorelin is available as 3.75 mg monthly dose and 11.25 mg three month dose. These formulations are considered equivalent in efficacy.

Side effects are from testosterone deprivation (hence, common to medical and surgical castration) and include sexual, such as impotence, loss of libido; metabolic, such as dyslipidemia including reduction in HDL-cholesterol with elevated cardiovascular risk; changes in body habitus due to fat distribution, gynecomastia, hair loss, loss of muscle mass, bone loss, hot flashes and night sweats. Bone loss is 3–5% in the first year of ADT and is associated with a higher incidence of osteoporotic fractures.

5.3.1.3 *Estrogens*

The Veterans Administrative groups conducted the initial trials with the non-steroidal estrogen, diethylstilbestrol (DES) that revealed a role in metastatic prostate cancer. DES inhibits LHRH release from the hypothalamus in addition to peripheral blockade of the androgen receptor and direct cytotoxic effects on the cancer cells. The VACURG studied the role of this agent in randomized trials in patients with advanced prostate cancer. Prostate cancer specific survival was better in patients receiving 1 mg DES. However, this benefit was offset by the markedly increased cardiovascular deaths with DES.

Estrogen use is complicated by marked cardiovascular toxicity due to thrombogenesis and to fluid retention, especially at the higher daily doses of ≥3 mg that correlate with consistent castrate testosterone levels. Conjugated estrogens, ethinyl estradiol and medroxyprogesterone acetate have been tested and are occasionally used in the second-line setting.

5.3.2 **Peripheral blockade**

5.3.2.1 *Anti-androgens*

These agents competitively block the androgen receptor (AR) in peripheral tissues such as the prostate. Because of feedback loops, with pure anti-androgens the serum testosterone levels rise rather than fall, obviating some of the toxicities of LHRH agonist therapy. The advantages with anti-androgens include oral administration and rapid immediate onset of activity. Non-steroidal options include flutamide, bicalutamide and nilutamide; the steroidal anti-androgen cyproterone acetate is used in Europe. Anti-androgens are generally not recommended as monotherapy because of a suggestion of inferior efficacy compared to LHRH agonist or surgical castration.

Administration and dosing: Flutamide has a short half-life of 5 hours and is dosed at 250 mg every 8 hours. Half-lives of bicalutamide and nilutamide are longer (approximately 5 days and 2 days) and are dosed once a day (bicalutamide as a single agent at usual daily dose of 150 mg).

Side effects: Gastrointestinal: nausea, vomiting, diarrhea and potentially fatal hepatotoxicity (least with bicalutamide but requires periodic liver function tests with use of any anti-androgen); breast growth or enlargement with or without tenderness. Nilutamide has, in addition, specific toxicities of decreased dark adaptation, rare but serious interstitial pneumonitis and alcohol intolerance. Sexual function is likely to be better preserved with pure anti-androgens compared to LHRH agonists.

5.3.2.2 *Other*

5-alpha reductase inhibitors have been used in conjunction with anti-androgens (so-called peripheral androgen blockade) and in addition to both LHRH agonist and anti-androgen (so-called triple androgen blockade). Currently, there is no convincing evidence for either of these approaches as primary therapy for new metastatic disease.

5.4 **Monitoring of ADT**

Monitoring of ADT involves periodically obtaining details of symptoms with particular attention to potential side effects, physical examination, PSA levels, and re-staging as necessitated by new symptoms or rapid changes in PSA. Preventive measures include periodic bone densitometry studies at onset and during treatment, calcium and vitamin D supplements, control of cardiac risk factors through exercise, dietary modification and medications, and symptom-directed management such as selective serotonin reuptake inhibitors (SSRI) for hot flashes. Gynaecomastia is rarely severe enough with LHRH agonists to warrant specific therapy (tamoxifen or other selective estrogen receptor modulators, aromatase inhibitors, surgery or prophylactic or therapeutic radiation).

5.5 Special considerations

5.5.1 Combined therapy versus monotherapy

The results of primary gonadal suppression + anti-androgen (CAB) versus monotherapy with primary gonadal suppression are shown in Table 5.1.

Adrenal androgens are thought to account for ~10% of the androgens driving prostate cancer. Orchiectomy or LHRH agonists ablate gonadal sources of androgens. Combined treatment with LHRH agonist and an anti-androgen has been attempted to improve duration and depth of responses. Results from several randomized trials have been conflicting in this regard (Table 5.1).

Three large meta-analyses have been conducted to address the issue. A Cochrane review pooled more than 6,000 patients from 20 trials comparing combined therapy with monotherapy including orchiectomy. At 5 years, odds ratio for overall survival favored CAB (1.29, 95% CI=1.11–1.5). Interestingly, the benefit was manifested earliest at 5 years. As expected, CAB had a more adverse toxicity profile. Samson et al reported the results of a meta-analysis comprising data from 21 trials and 6,871 patients. At 5 years of follow-up, HR for death for the CAB group was 0.87 (95% CI= 0.805–0.942). Interpretation was rendered difficult by the fact that only 10 of the 21 studies had 5-year survival data, the earliest time point at which CAB showed a survival advantage.

The Prostate Cancer Trialists' Collaborative Group (PCTCG) meta-analysis was published in 2000. Individual patient data from 8,275 men in 27 randomized trials were re-analyzed. 88% of patients had metastatic prostate cancer. 5-year survival was 25.4% with CAB versus 23.6% with monotherapy alone (p = 0.11). There was no significant heterogeneity in the treatment effect (MAB vs AS) with respect to age or disease stage. Data from patients who received nilutamide and flutamide (~80% of the patients), rather than cyproterone acetate, favored CAB (p = 0.005). Non-prostate-cancer deaths (although not clearly significantly affected by treatment) accounted for some of the apparently adverse effects of cyproterone acetate.

Result	Trial	N	Arm A	Arm B	Outcomes (A vs B)
	INT 0036 (USA)	603	Leuprolide + flutamide	Leuprolide + flutamide	PFS 17 m v 14 m*; mOS 36 m v 28 m*
	EORTC 30853	297	Goserelin + flutamide	Orchiec-tomy	Improved OS* (P = .04), TTP* (P=.009) and PFS* (P=.02)
Favouring CAB	Anandtron Study Group	457	Orchiec-tomy + nilutamide	Orchiec-tomy + placebo	TTP 21 m v 15 m*
	Japanese Trial	205	GnRH agonist + bicalutamide	GnRH agonist alone	mOS 37 m v 30 m; Improved TTF 117 v 60 weeks* and TTP (P < .001)
	INT 0105 (USA)	1387	Orchiec-tomy	Orchiec-tomy + flutamide	TTP: 20.4 m v 18.6 m mOS: 34 m v 30 m
Not favouring CAB	Danish Prostatic Cancer Group Trial 86	264	Goserelin + flutamide	Goserelin alone	OS, cause-specific survival, TTP not differrent
	Canadian Trial	208	Orchiec-tomy + nilutamide	Orchiec-tomy + placebo	TTP and OS not sig. different

Table 5.1 Randomized trials of combined treatment with an LHRH agonist and an anti-androgen

CAB–combined androgen blockade; OS–overall survival; PFS–progression free survival; TTF–time to treatment failure; TTP–time to progression; * Significant.

Using the delta method, another group studied data from an earlier meta-analysis of trials of CAB containing nilutamide and flutamide by the PCTCG and an additional trial containing bicalutamide. A significant benefit to CAB (orchiectomy and bicalutamide), a 20% reduction in death (95% CI = 2–34%) was seen.

Based on the PTCGC meta-analysis, it is estimated that CAB (with a non-steroidal anti-androgen) probably has a 2–3% absolute benefit in survival over monotherapy with LHRH agonist. At the present time, a decision on CAB will need to be made for each individual patient with due consideration of likely benefit, increased toxicities, and costs of therapy.

5.5.2 Early versus late ADT

The customary approach is to implement therapy at time of development of metastases. To address the question of timing of therapy; early therapy at diagnosis versus therapy at time of symptomatic disease, the Medical Research Council (MRC) in the UK performed a randomized phase III trial. 938 patients with locally advanced or asymptomatic metastatic disease were randomized to immediate ADT (medical/surgical castration) versus deferred therapy to begin at onset of symptoms/other indications. 361 men died in the deferred therapy arm versus 328 in the immediate ADT arm (p = 0.02). The rate of death from prostate cancer favoured the immediate therapy arm (203 or 62% versus 257 or 71% in the deferred; p = 0.001). Disease related complications such as pathologic skeletal fractures, development of overt and painful metastases, and cord compression occurred twice as commonly in the deferred therapy arm (for cord compression, 5% versus 2%, p <0.025). These data support the use of early therapy at diagnosis to avoid disease related complications. Criticisms of the MRC trial include lack of accurate staging by bone scans, heterogeneity in follow-up schedules at the discretion of the physician, lack of any hormone treatment in some of the men, and failure to complete target accrual.

5.5.3 **Continuous versus intermittent ADT**

ADT is associated with adverse effects and impact on quality of life. Furthermore virtually all patients with metastatic disease will progress despite androgen deprivation. Based on preclinical data, intermittent androgen deprivation therapy attempts to delay the emergence of androgen independence while potentially minimizing toxicities. Data from phase II studies suggested intermittent ADT is a feasible option. A recently completed large multicenter international SWOG lead trial (S9346) is comparing survival of continuous versus intermittent androgen deprivation specifically in patients with new M1 prostate cancer. Although intermittent ADT can be considered in selected patients, its wide use application is considered experimental pending the results of the phase III trial.

5.6 **Changes in PSA levels as prognostic markers**

Data from SWOG study 9346 showed that lower the PSA at the end of 7 months of ADT, the better the overall survival. Patients with a PSA of ≤ 4 ng/mL had less than one third the risk of death as those with a PSA of > 4 ng/mL (P < .001). The median survival for the two groups was 68 months and 16 months respectively. Additionally, patients with PSA of ≤ 0.2 ng/mL had less than one fifth the risk of death as patients with a PSA of > 4 ng/mL (P < .001). Moreover, those with a PSA ≤ 0.2 ng/mL had significantly improved survival than those with PSA of > 0.2 to 4 ng/mL (p < .001). Median survival was 13 months for patients with a PSA of > 4 ng/mL, 44 months for patients with PSA of greater than 0.2 to 4 ng/mL, and 75 months for patients with PSA of ≤ 0.2 ng/mL.

A recent secondary analysis has demonstrated that patients with PSA progression, defined as a 25% increase in PSA levels with absolute value $\geq$ 2ng/mL, had a significantly increased risk of death (HR 2.49; 95% CI = 2.09–2.85; p<0.0001) in the continuous arm of SWOG 9346 trial (1078 patients analyzed). Similarly, the median survival for those with PSA progression as defined above was 10 months compared to 44 months for those without PSA progression.

Further reading

Bhandari MS, Crook J, Hussain M (2005). Should intermittent androgen deprivation be used in routine clinical practice? *J Clin Oncol*, **23**(32), 8212–8.

Crawford ED, Eisenberger MA, McLeod DG, Spaulding JT, Benson R, Dorr FA, Blumenstein BA, Davis MA, Goodman PJ (1989). A controlled trial of leuprolide with and without flutamide in prostatic carcinoma. *N Engl J Med*, **321**(7), 419–24. Erratum in: *N Engl J Med* (1989) **321**(20), 1420.

El-Rayes BF, Hussain MH (2002). Hormonal therapy for prostate cancer: past, present and future. *Expert Review of Anticancer Therapy*, **2**(1), 37–47.

Klotz L, Schellhammer P, Carroll K (2004). A re-assessment of the role of combined androgen blockade for advanced prostate cancer, **93**(9), 1177–82.

Medical Research Council Trial. The Medical Research Council Prostate Cancer Working Party Investigators Group; no authors listed (1997). Immediate versus deferred treatment for advanced prostatic cancer: initial results of the *Br J Urol.*, **79**(2), 235–46.

Hussain M, Tangen CM, Higano C, Schelhammer PF, Faulkner J, Crawford ED, Wilding G, Akdas A, Small EJ, Donnelly B, MacVicar G, Raghavan D; Southwest Oncology Group Trial 9346 (INT-0162) (2006). Absolute prostate-specific antigen value after androgen deprivation is a strong independent predictor of survival in new metastatic prostate cancer: Data from Southwest Oncology Group Trial 9346 (INT-0162), **24**(24), 3984–90.

Prostate Cancer Trialists' Collaborative Group; Maximum androgen blockade in advanced prostate cancer: an overview of the randomised trials (2000). *Lancet*, **355**(9214), 1491–8.

Samson DJ, Seidenfeld J, Schmitt B, Hasselblad V, Albertsen PC, Bennett CL, Wilt TJ (2002). Systematic review and meta-analysis of monotherapy compared with combined androgen blockade for patients with advanced prostate carcinoma. *Cancer*, **95**(2), 361–76.

Seidenfeld J, Samson DJ, Hasselblad V, Aronson N, Albertsen PC, Bennett CL, Wilt TJ (2000). Single-therapy androgen suppression in men with advanced prostate cancer: a systematic review and meta-analysis. *Ann Intern Med.*, **132**(7), 566–77.

Schmitt B, Bennett C, Seidenfeld J, Samson D, Wilt T (2000). Maximal androgen blockade for advanced prostate cancer. *Cochrane Database Syst Rev.*, (2):CD001526.

Chapter 6

Second- and third-line hormone therapies

Wolfgang Lilleby and Sophie Fosså

Key points

- Castration-refractory prostate cancer (CRPC) is defined as progression despite ongoing primary androgen deprivation therapy
- Paradoxical androgen receptor stimulation can be seen and will respond to anti-androgen withdrawal
- Steroids offer only limitedly-effective second-line therapy and one has to be aware of side effects
- Selective blocking of cytochrome P17 with abiraterone opens a novel treatment option but is still an experimental approach.

6.1 Pathways of progression during androgen deprivation therapy

In 70–80% of patients with newly diagnosed prostate cancer the growth and survival of most malignant cells depend on the 5 alpha-reduced metabolite of testosterone (5 alpha-dihydrotestosterone) and a functioning androgen receptor. Androgen suppression therapy (ADT) is followed by castration levels of serum testosterone (<20ng/dL) and leads to objective and subjective remission. Depending on the differentiation of the primary lesion and the tumor burden, the median time to clinical progression is 3–5 years after start of ADT overall, and 1–2 years in patients treated for metastatic disease.

Progression of PC during ADT is believed to occur along two different pathways. Malignant cell clones may develop which no longer need functioning androgen receptors for their growth and survival, but are dependent on oncogenically acting proteins, for example, BCL2, neuropeptides, insulin-like growth factors or other signaling pathways. These cells are refractory to any hormone influences. (Castration Refractory Prostate cancer [CRPC].)

The development along the other pathway ends with prostate cancer cells which are hypersensitive to androgenic influences. During ADT the androgen receptors in the cancer cell can be amplified or mutated, leading to hypersensitivity to very low residual androgens in the serum. Such cells are sensitive to pharmacologically induced changes in the hormone milieu (Figure 6.1). Second- and third-line treatment of prostate cancer has to be based on the understanding of these developmental steps of prostate malignancy.

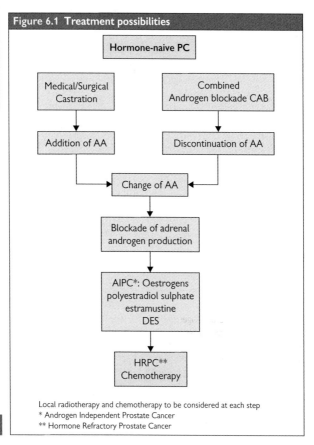

Figure 6.1 Treatment possibilities

Local radiotherapy and chemotherapy to be considered at each step
* Androgen Independent Prostate Cancer
** Hormone Refractory Prostate Cancer

Patients progressing during ADT have been treated either by medical or surgical castration alone or they have had long-lasting combined androgen blockade (CAB) (medical or surgical castration + anti-androgen (AA). Further treatment is guided by the type of the initial ADT. Importantly ADT should be continued indefinitely to suppress growth of the remaining sensitive hormone cells.

6.2 Anti-androgen withdrawal

In patients with initial CAB the anti-androgen (Flutamide, bicalutamide, nilutamide) should be discontinued as a first step as this drug may have androgenic function in cells with an amplified or mutated AR gene. Such anti-androgen withdrawal leads to PSA decrease in 20–30% of the patients. The biochemical duration of this intervention may last up to 5 months. No survival benefit has been demonstrated.

6.3 Anti-androgen addition

In patients progressing on surgical or medical castration alone as first line ADT the addition of an anti-androgen leads to PSA responses in 20–30% of the patients with a favourable toxicity profile. Side-effects of flutamide are diarrhoea and skin hyper-reactivity to the sun. Both flutamide and bicalutamide may result in increase of serum liver function tests in up to 30% of the patients. When PSA is rising again the clinician should stop the anti-androgen, or consider changing the anti-androgen. There have been secondary responses to high-dose bicalutamide in patients, who progressed on flutamide.

6.4 Suppression of adrenal androgen production

The adrenal glands produce low levels of androgens which may stimulate amplified or mutated androgen receptors. Inhibition of the production of these steroids may consequently lead to remission of progressive PC. In America the preferred drug is ketoconazole. About 50% of the patients will experience PSA declines during such treatment. High-dose ketoconazole therapy has to be combined with hydrocortisone. In Europe, most often prednisolone 10–20 mg per day or dexamethasone 0.5 mg per day has been used with PSA responses in about 20% of the patients and occasionally with objective responses. The introduction of abiraterone represents a further development in the attempt to inhibit androgen production and thereby suppress the androgenic supply to the cancer cells. Abiraterone is a selective inhibitor of cytochrome P17, which is necessary for the production of dihydro-epi-androstenedione and androstenedione. In a phase I study 12 of 21 patients most of them on prior treatment with dexamethasone experienced PSA reduction of ≥50%, with occasional objective remissions and improved symptoms. Toxicity consisted of hypertension, hypokalemia and oedema (excess of mineralocorticoid).

6.5 **Estrogens**

Both prostate cancer cells and the surrounding non-cancer tissue express estrogens receptors, though their role for cellular growth is unknown. Nevertheless, clinical experience has shown that PSA reductions can be achieved in up to 50% of the patients by small oral doses of diethylstilbestrol (DES), 1 mg daily. Estramustine is another predominantly estrogenic agent, which has been used in prostate cancer patients progressing on ADT, however, with an increased risk of thrombosis and cardiovascular complications. Transdermal estrogen therapy is experimental.

6.6 **Conclusion**

Secondary hormonal manipulation is an accepted and clinically worthwhile approach to achieve PSA reduction, symptom relief and occasionally objective responses in up to one third of patients progressing on ADT. However, no survival benefit has been shown for any of the available treatment modalities. Therefore, chemotherapy, recently shown to be capable of prolonging life, should also be considered when starting secondary hormone treatment.

Further reading

Attard G, Reid A, et al. (2008). Phase I clinical trial of a selective inhibitor of CYP17. JCO, **26**(28), 4563–71.

Debes JD, Tindall DJ (2004). Mechanisms of androgen-refractory prostate cancer. NEJM, **315**(15), 1488–90.

Figg W, Sartor O, Cooper ME, et al. (1995). Prostate-specific antigen decline following the discontinuation of flutamide in patients with stage D2 prostate cancer. Am J Med, **98**, 412–14.

Fossa SD, Slee PH, Brausi M, et al. (2001). Flutamide versus prednisone in patients with prostate cancer symptomatically progressing after androgen-ablative therapy: a phase 111 study of the European organisation for research and treatment of cancergenitourinary group. JCO, **19**, 62–71.

Small EJ, Halabi S, Dawson NA, et al. (2004). Antiandrogen withdrawal alone or in combination with ketoconazole in androgen-independent prostate cancer patients: A phase III trial (CALGB 9583). JCO, **22**, 1025–33.

Smith DC et al. (1998). A phase 11 trial of oral stilboestrol as a second-line hormonal agent in advanced prostate cancer. Urology, **52**, 257–60.

Chapter 7

Chemotherapy for metastatic prostate cancer

Cora N Sternberg and Guru Sonpavde

Key points

- Docetaxel-based chemotherapy has been shown to modestly extend life, relieve pain, and improve the quality of life in patients with metastatic castration-resistant prostate cancer
- Current trials are attempting to build on the backbone of docetaxel by combining it with novel biologic agents
- Trials are also investigating the role of docetaxel for earlier stages of prostate cancer
- No standard second-line chemotherapy exists and such patients are candidates for trials. The increased understanding of the mechanisms of progressive castration-resistant prostate cancer is being translated into an increasing pipeline of novel therapies.

7.1 Introduction

While metastatic prostate cancer almost always responds to initial androgen deprivation therapy (ADT), the disease universally progresses to a phase when ADT alone fails to control the malignancy despite castrate testosterone levels. This phase of the disease is termed castration-resistant prostate cancer (CRPC). The earlier terms 'androgen independent' or 'hormone-refractory' prostate cancer have been increasingly discarded since a proportion of patients continue to depend on the androgen axis and may respond to second and third-line hormonal manipulations. CRPC comprises patients with diverse clinical subtypes including a rising PSA (prostate specific antigen) alone or with metastases, radiological progression (bone scan, nodal, or visceral progression) and clinical progression (worsening pain, urinary

obstruction, spinal cord compression). By convention, ADT is continued in patients with CRPC, in order to maintain castrate testosterone
levels. Until the emergence of docetaxel chemotherapy, effective
agents that objectively improved outcomes were not available for
metastatic CRPC. This review discusses the current management of
metastatic CRPC with systemic chemotherapy.

7.2 Mitoxantrone chemotherapy: palliative benefits only

Mitoxantrone chemotherapy was evaluated in a two key randomized
phase III clinical trials performed in the mid-1990s (Table 7.1).
Rather than traditional survival and response criteria, the trial by
Tannock and colleagues primarily evaluated palliative endpoints. The
trial randomized 161 symptomatic metastatic CRPC patients (with
pain) to prednisone 5 mg twice daily versus mitoxantrone 12 mg/m^2
every 3 weeks plus prednisone 5 mg twice daily (MP). To mitigate
cardiac toxicities, patients who were still responding after a cumulative dose of 140 mg/m^2 of mitoxantrone continued treatment with
prednisone alone. Progression was defined as an increase in the
present pain intensity (PPI) scale of 1 point compared with the nadir
or an increase in analgesic score of >25% compared with baseline,
each maintained on two consecutive visits. Unequivocal evidence of
radiologic progression or a requirement for radiation therapy also
constituted disease progression. Palliative response defined by a ≥ 2
point decline in pain on the 6-point McGill pain questionnaire was
the major endpoint. Palliative response occurred significantly more
often with MP compared to prednisone alone (29% vs. 12%, P<.01).

Table 7.1 Reported key randomized phase III chemotherapy trials for metastatic CRPC					
Author (reference)	N	Setting	Control group	Experimental group	Improved survival
Tannock	161	1st-line	P	MP	No, improved QOL
Kantoff	242	1st-line	H	MH	No, improved PFS
Tannock	1006	1st-line	MP	DP	Yes
Petrylak	770	1st-line	MP	EMP-Docetaxel	Yes
Sternberg	950	2nd-line	P	Satraplatin-P	No, improved PFS

N—number of patients; P—prednisone; MP—mitoxantrone/prednisone; QOL—quality of life;
H—hydrocortisone; MH—mitoxantrone/hydrocortisone; PFS—progression free survival;
DP—3-weekly docetaxel/prednisone; EMP—estramustine phosphate.

In addition, a significantly longer duration of response of 43 weeks versus 18 weeks (P = <.001) was also attained. Overall survival was not different with a median survival of approximately 1 year in both groups, potentially a result of the crossover design, or the small number of patients conferring limited power. Eleven of 50 patients randomized to prednisone treatment responded after addition of mitoxantrone. Palliative response correlated incompletely with a decrease in serum PSA level. Among all 130 patients who received mitoxantrone (including crossover), 5 patients who received cumulative doses of 116 to 214 mg/m^2 developed cardiac dysfunction. Two of these 5 patients exhibited symptomatic congestive heart failure, but none died of cardiac causes. There were only 9 instances of neutropenic fever among 130 patients who received mitoxantrone, and alopecia and severe emesis were rare.

The second trial, CALGB-9182, accrued 242 patients and had a primary endpoint of overall survival. Similar patients with metastatic CRPC were accrued, except that pain was not a requirement. This trial utilized hydrocortisone 30 mg in the morning and 10 mg in the afternoon with or without mitoxantrone 14 mg/m^2 every 3 weeks, and crossover was not permitted. Again, overall survival was not significantly different with a median of approximately 1 year. The duration of response with chemotherapy was significantly longer (3.7 months vs. 2.3 months, P = 0.025) and some improvement in pain control was also observed. Cardiac dysfunction and neutropenic infections were rare with mitoxantrone therapy. These studies established mitoxantrone chemotherapy as a viable option for palliative treatment in patients with metastatic CRPC.

7.3 Docetaxel based chemotherapy: survival and palliative benefits

Based on encouraging PSA response rates as well as survival data in early trials of docetaxel alone or in combination with estramustine phosphate (EMP), randomized studies were conducted comparing docetaxel-based therapy with MP (Table 7.1). In the phase III TAX-327 study, two schedules of docetaxel were compared with the standard mitoxantrone regimen (12 mg/m^2 every 3 weeks), with all patients receiving prednisone. This was the largest randomized trial in metastatic CRPC to date with 1,006 patients accrued. Patients with brain or leptomeningeal metastases and peripheral neuropathy ≥grade 2 were excluded. The weekly regimen consisted of docetaxel 30 mg/m^2 every week for 5 of 6 weeks and the every 3 week regimen consisted of docetaxel 75 mg/m^2 every 3 weeks. Patients in all arms received prednisone 5 mg twice a day. Therapy was administered until progressive disease and up to a maximum of 10 cycles for the groups given docetaxel every 3 weeks or mitoxantrone and up to 5 cycles (of 6 weeks each) in the weekly-docetaxel group. Progressive disease was defined as pain progression (defined as an increase in the PPI score of ≥1 point from the nadir, an increase in the analgesic score of ≥25%, or a requirement for palliative radiotherapy), PSA progression (defined as an increase from the nadir of either ≥25% for men with no PSA response or ≥50% for all others) or objective progression of measurable disease. Pain response was defined as a reduction in the PPI score of ≥2 points from baseline without an increase in the analgesic score or as a reduction of ≥50% in the analgesic score without an increase in the PPI score, either of which was maintained for ≥3 weeks. In an update of this study, median survival was 19.2 months in the 3-week docetaxel group, 17.8 months with weekly docetaxel, and 16.3 months with mitoxantrone. The 3-year survivals were 17.9%, 16.7% and 13.7%, respectively. Only 3-week docetaxel plus prednisone attained statistical superiority when compared to MP. The survival benefit of docetaxel given every three weeks was consistent across subgroups defined according to the presence or absence of pain, Karnofsky performance-status score (≤70 vs. ≥80) and age (<65 years vs. ≥65 years). Measurable tumor response rates were low and comparable in all arms. More patients in the 3-week docetaxel arm experienced a significant reduction in pain compared to mitoxantrone (35% vs. 22%, P = 0.01). Nearly a quarter of patients in each docetaxel arm (22% with 3-week and 23% with weekly) exhibited a significant improvement in quality of life compared with mitoxantrone (13%). PSA response rate was better in each docetaxel arm: 45% with every-3-weeks administration and 48% with weekly administration versus 32% with mitoxantrone. Grade 3/4 neutropenia occurred in 32% of patients treated with every-3-weekly docetaxel, 22% treated with mitoxantrone, and only 1.5% treated with weekly docetaxel. However, febrile neutropenia and infection were uncommon in all groups (0–3%), and there were no septic deaths. There was a higher incidence of grade 3–4 cardiac dysfunction among patients who received mitoxantrone compared to both docetaxel groups (7% vs. 1–2%). Docetaxel induced more fatigue, alopecia, diarrhea, nail changes, sensory neuropathy, anorexia, changes in taste, stomatitis, dyspnea, tearing, peripheral edema, and epistaxis. Most adverse events associated with docetaxel were low grade and not life-threatening, with loss of sensation in the fingers and toes being particularly annoying to some patients. However, the overall outcomes suggest that docetaxel has superior palliative effects despite the increase in toxicity.

In the Southwest Oncology Group (SWOG)-9916 phase III trial, 770 patients with metastatic CRPC were randomized to combination docetaxel-EMP or MP. Patients were ineligible if they had received rior radioisotope or anticoagulant therapy (excluding aspirin), had active thrombophlebitis, hypercoagulability or a history of pulmonary embolus. Patients in the docetaxel-EMP group received docetaxel 60 mg/m^2 every 3 weeks plus 5 consecutive days of EMP 280 mg given orally for 3 times a day. Patients in the MP group received mitoxantrone 12 mg/m^2 every 3 weeks plus continuous prednisone at a dose of 5 mg twice a day. Patients who did not experience grade 3/4 toxicity in the first cycle of therapy had the docetaxel dose escalated to 70 mg/m^2 or the mitoxantrone dose escalated to 14 mg/m^2. With studies demonstrating the utility of prophylactic anticoagulation in decreasing EMP-related vascular events, the protocol was amended to include daily warfarin (2 mg) and aspirin (325 mg) in the docetaxel-EMP group. Treatment continued until disease progression or unacceptable adverse effects occurred or until a maximum of 12 cycles of docetaxel-EMP or 144 mg/m^2 of mitoxantrone had been administered. Progression was defined as objective or PSA progression ($\geq$25% and $\geq$ 5 ng/ml increase in the serum PSA over the last pre-registration or nadir measurement, with confirmation of the increase at least 4 weeks later) or death. The median survival was significantly improved with the docetaxel-EMP combination (17.5 vs. 15.6 months, P = 0.02), the relative risk of death was reduced by 20% and the PSA response rate was significantly better (50% vs. 27%, P <0.001). The median time to progression was 6.3 months for docetaxel-EMP and 3.2 months for MP (P<0.001). Greater toxicity was observed in the docetaxel-EMP group: grade 3/4 gastrointestinal (20% vs. 5%), hematologic (neutropenic fever, 5% vs. 2%), cardiovascular (15% vs. 7%), metabolic disturbances (6% vs. 1%), and neurologic events (7% vs. 2%) were all more frequent in the docetaxel-EMP arm.

Clearly, significant improvements in overall survival and palliative benefits were demonstrated with the 3-week docetaxel based regimen, establishing it as the cornerstone of frontline systemic chemotherapy for metastatic CRPC. Weekly docetaxel may be considered in more frail patients, given the demonstration of palliative benefits and lower myelosuppression. EMP is associated with significant gastrointestinal and thromboembolic toxicities that have led to decreased usage. Given the toxicities attributable to EMP and the similar benefit with docetaxel plus prednisone and docetaxel plus EMP, the combination of docetaxel plus prednisone has been approved by regulatory authorities and has become the preferred regimen for the frontline treatment of metastatic CRPC. Ongoing phase III trials are attempting to improve upon the benefits of docetaxel by combining it with novel biologic agents (e.g. bevacizumab, aflibercept, dasatinib, ZD4054, atrasentan, anti-clusterin etc.).

7.4 **Second-line chemotherapy following docetaxel**

Effective salvage therapy following prior docetaxel is lacking, as only modest and similar efficacy has been demonstrated with mitoxantrone or ixabepilone in this setting. In a randomized phase II trial comparing mitoxantrone plus prednisone with ixabepilone without prednisone in patients progressing after docetaxel, the median time to progression was approximately 2.2 months, the median survival was 10.4 months with ixabepilone and 9.8 months with MP, and ≥50% PSA declines were noted in 17% of ixabepilone and 20% of MP patients. Satraplatin is a third-generation orally available platinum analog which demonstrated a 33% reduction in the risk of progression or death in patients with metastatic CRPC following one prior chemotherapy regimen in the 950 patient phase III SPARC (Satraplatin and Prednisone Against Refractory Cancer) trial. Satraplatin also demonstrated beneficial effects on pain and biologic activity with PSA declines and objective responses. Unfortunately, satraplatin did not significantly extend survival (median survival of approximately 13 months in both groups), although this analysis might have been confounded by post-study therapy. Therefore, approval by regulatory agencies has not been granted. Given the dismal outcomes with currently available second-line agents, patients with progressive metastatic CRPC following docetaxel-based chemotherapy are excellent candidates for clinical trials.

7.5 **Metastatic CRPC with neuroendocrine differentiation: recognition and treatment**

Small-cell neuroendocrine carcinoma of the prostate is a rare histological variant occurring in 0.5% to 2.0% of prostatic primary tumors. This phenotype may be more common in the castration-resistant state. One should evaluate for neuroendocrine differentiation with a biopsy in those with advanced stage, but relatively low serum PSA. These tumors may secrete neuroendocrine markers such as neuron-specific enolase or chromogrannin A, or adrenocorticotropic hormone or antidiuretic hormone. Therapy for advanced small-cell carcinomas of the prostate is extrapolated from therapy for small-cell carcinomas of the lung, and the combination of a platinum and etoposide is considered the conventional regimen.

7.6 **Prognostic factors in patients with metastatic CRPC**

Ten independent prognostic factors were identified in a multivariate analysis of the TAX-327 trial: liver metastases, number of metastatic sites, significant pain, Karnofsky performance status, type of progression (measurable disease or bone scan progression), pretreatment PSA-doubling time (DT), absolute PSA level, tumor grade, alkaline phosphatase, and hemoglobin. These factors have been incorporated into a nomogram, which may be useful for stratification in future clinical trials, however further validation of this nomogram is necessary.

7.7 **Surrogate endpoints for response and progression**

Prostate cancer is characterized by a poor ability to measure response and progression due either to immeasurable bone-only metastases or PSA-only disease. Optimal surrogate endpoints for measuring the status of disease-burden are lacking. PSA response has historically been defined as a ≥50% decline. However, a PSA decline of ≥30% at 3 months appears to be a more useful, albeit imperfect, intermediate surrogate for improved long-term outcomes with cytotoxic chemotherapy. Data from the TAX-327 trial were employed to analyze PSA declines ranging from 0% to 90%, PSA velocity and pain response as intermediate surrogate end-points. A PSA decline of ≥30% within 3 months of chemotherapy initiation had the highest degree of surrogacy for overall survival. Other changes in PSA, PSA kinetics, PSA normalization, and pain responses were weaker surrogates for survival. A similar retrospective analysis of the SWOG-9916 trial analyzed PSA velocity and PSA declines ranging from 5% to 90% within 3 months for surrogacy. The optimal biochemical surrogate was again found to be a ≥30% PSA decline. A recent analysis by SWOG suggests that a ≥25% PSA increase at 3 months may be a useful surrogate for poor survival in patients with metastatic CRPC. Alternatively, time to event endpoints may be clinically useful surrogates, can be employed to make clinical decisions, and are currently recommended in the setting of clinical trials by the prostate cancer working group (PCWG)-2 guidelines. In particular, progression-free survival defined as a composite endpoint constituted by symptomatic or radiologic progression may be a clinically relevant endpoint and preliminarily appears to be a useful intermediate surrogate for survival in the setting of frontline chemotherapy. Recent and ongoing trials are frequently defining bone progression as the presence of ≥2 new lesions confirmed by further new lesions on repeat bone scanning after ≥4 weeks. Other useful intermediate surrogates are emerging, such as an early change of CTCs (circulating tumor cells) All of these intermediate surrogates for outcomes require prospective validation.

7.8 Chemotherapy for earlier stages of prostate cancer

The application of chemotherapy to earlier stages of prostate cancer is investigational. Chemotherapy is not accepted as standard for patients with non-metastatic CRPC with PSA-only disease. A multitude of trials are evaluating the role of early chemotherapy (Table 7.2). Randomized trials are evaluating the benefit of adding docetaxel to ADT for metastatic and/or non-metastatic castration-sensitive prostate cancer (STAMPEDE and CHAARTED trials). Trials are ongoing for patients with non-metastatic prostate cancer with high risk features such as PSA ≥ 20 ng/mL, Gleason ≥ 8, T2c disease or rapid PSA-doubling following local therapy, and following combination radiation and ADT. Unfortunately, adjuvant mitoxantrone therapy following radical prostatectomy for high-risk localized prostate cancer induced an increase in acute leukemia. Another trial that was comparing adjuvant versus delayed ADT with or without docetaxel was terminated prematurely due to poor accrual. Separate randomized trials in the U.S. Veterans Affairs hospital system and Sweden are evaluating the role of adjuvant docetaxel alone without ADT for patients with high-risk localized prostate cancer following radical prostatectomy. Both the Radiation therapy Oncology Group and a Finnish trial are evaluating docetaxel and ADT versus ADT alone after radiation therapy (RT) in high risk locally advanced patients. Combination docetaxel and ADT prior to local therapy (surgery or RT) is being evaluated by several groups (Table 7.2).

7.9 Conclusions

Docetaxel-based chemotherapy has both extended survival and provided palliative benefits for patients with metastatic CRPC. However, the benefits are modest, and efforts are ongoing to further improve outcomes by combining docetaxel with novel biologic agents. Novel agents are being evaluated in clinical trials for progressive disease following docetaxel since no effective therapeutics exist for these patients. Additionally, the role of chemotherapy for earlier stages of prostate cancer is being evaluated. Further advances are possible by an improved understanding of the biology of prostate cancer and rational drug development.

Table 7.2 Ongoing phase III trials evaluating chemotherapy for earlier stages of prostate cancer

Institution	Setting	Control therapy	Experimental therapy
U.S. Intergroup (CHAARTED)	Metastatic CSPC	ADT	ADT + D
European (STAMPEDE)	Metastatic or non-metastatic CSPC	ADT	ADT + D[#]
Multicenter TAX-3503 trial	Non-metastatic CSPC with PSADT ≤ 9 months	ADT	ADT + D
RTOG, Finnish*	Locally advanced prostate cancer	RT + ADT→ ADT	XRT + ADT → ADT + (D + P)
U.S. Veterans Affairs, Swedish*	Localized high-risk prostate cancer	Prostatectomy	Prostatectomy → D
U.S. Intergroup	Localized high-risk prostate cancer	Prostatectomy	ADT + D → Prostatectomy
NCIC	Localized high-risk prostate cancer	ADT → RT + ADT	D + ADT → RT + ADT
DFCI	Localized intermediate/ high-risk prostate cancer	ADT → RT	D + ADT → RT
European (GETUG)	Localized high-risk prostate cancer	ADT → Prostatectomy/RT	ADT + (D + EMP) → Prostatectomy/RT

[#] Experimental arms also include ADT combined with one of the following treatments: zoledronic acid, celecoxib, celecoxib plus zoledronic acid, docetaxel plus zoledronic acid; * separate trials; CSPC- castration sensitive prostate cancer; ADT- androgen deprivation therapy; D- docetaxel; P- prednisone; RTOG- Radiation Therapy Oncology Group; RT- radiation therapy; NCIC- National Cancer Institute of Canada; RT- radiation therapy; DFCI- Dana Farber Cancer Institute; EMP- estramustine phosphate

57

Further reading

Armstrong AJ, Garrett-Mayer E, Yang YC, et al. (2007). A contemporary prognostic nomogram for men with hormone-refractory metastatic prostate cancer: a TAX327 study analysis. *Clin Cancer Res*, **13**(21), 6396–403.

Armstrong AJ, Garrett-Mayer E, Yang YC, et al. (2007) Prostate-specific antigen and pain surrogacy analysis in metastatic hormone-refractory prostate cancer. *J Clin Oncol*, **25**(25), 3965–70.

Berthold DR, Pond GR, Soban F, *et al.* (2008). Docetaxel plus prednisone or mitoxantrone plus prednisone for advanced prostate cancer: Updated survival of the TAX 327 study. *J Clin Oncol*, **26**(2), 242–45.

Kantoff PW, Halabi S, Conaway M, *et al.* (1999) Hydrocortisone with or without mitoxantrone in men with hormone-refractory prostate cancer: results of the cancer and leukemia group B 9182 study. *J Clin Oncol*, **17**(8), 2506–13.

Petrylak DP, Ankerst DP, Joang CS, *et al.* (2006) Evaluation of prostate-specific antigen declines for surrogacy in patients treated on SWOG 99–16. *J Natl Cancer Inst*, **98**(8), 516–21.

Petrylak DP, Tangen CM, Hussain MH, *et al.* Docetaxel and estramustine compared with mitoxantrone and prednisone for advanced refractory prostate cancer. *N Engl J Med*, **351**(15), 1513–20.

Rosenberg JE, Weinberg VK, Kelly WK, *et al.* (2007) Activity of second-line chemotherapy in docetaxel-refractory hormone-refractory prostate cancer patients: randomized phase 2 study of ixabepilone or mitoxantrone and prednisone. *Cancer*, **110**(3), 556–63.

Scher HI, Halabi S, Tannock I, *et al.* (2008) Design and end points of clinical trials for patients with progressive prostate cancer and castrate levels of testosterone: recommendations of the Prostate Cancer Clinical Trials Working Group. *J Clin Oncol*, **26**(7), 1148–59.

Sternberg CN, Petrylak D, Witjes F, *et al.* (2007) Satraplatin (S) demonstrates significant clinical benefits for the treatment of patients with HRPC: Results of a randomized phase III trial. *J Clin Oncol*, ASCO Annual Meeting Proceedings Part I. Vol 25, No. 18S (June 20 Supplement), 5019.

Tannock IF, Osoba D, Stockler MR, *et al.* (1996) Chemotherapy with mitoxantrone plus prednisone or prednisone alone for symptomatic hormone-resistant prostate cancer: a Canadian randomized trial with palliative end points. *J Clin Oncol*, **14**(6), 1756–64.

Chapter 8

The role of bisphosphonates in the systemic treatment of prostate cancer

Alan Horwich and David P Dearnaley

> **Key points**
> - Bone metastases are a major cause of morbidity in metastatic prostate cancer
> - Bisphosphonates have shown evidence of activity in inhibiting osteoclasts and in reducing the incidence of skeletal-related events in patients with bone metastases
> - Bisphosphonates may aid pain control in some patients with castrate resistant symptomatic bone metastases
> - Bisphosphonates moderate and reverse bone density loss associated with androgen suppression
> - There are significant side effect risks from long-term use of potent intravenous bisphosphonates including osteonecrosis of the jaw
> - The use of bisphosphonates should be considered in patients with prostate cancer at high risk of a skeletal related event
> - Ongoing clinical trials will further define the role of bisphosphonates in prostate cancer.

8.1 Introduction

Bone metastases are the predominant pattern of spread of metastatic prostate cancer and a major cause of morbidity including pain, pathological fracture, bone marrow failure, and spinal cord and nerve root compression syndromes. Hypercalcaemia is very uncommon. Metastases typically show an osteoblastic radiological pattern and most lesions are in the axial skeleton with relative sparing of the limbs, especially peripherally. It is thought that factors released by tumour cells stimulate both osteoclasts and osteoblasts, and in turn growth factors secreted by these cells can stimulate tumour growth. In the osteoblastic metastases there is an increase in both osteoblast and osteoclast numbers and activity with excess new bone formation and disorganisation of bone structure.

Bisphosphonates are synthetic analogues of pyrophosphate which are relatively resistant to hydrolysis. They bind preferentially to bone surfaces which are undergoing active remodelling and there they inhibit osteoclast maturation and suppress osteoclast functions. They also inhibit the recruitment of osteoclasts to these areas. There are a range of bisphosphonates whose potency assessed in vivo varies considerably. Clodronate and etidronate have relatively low potency, pamidronate and alendronate have intermediate potency and ibandronate and zoledronic acid are amongst the most potent drugs in their class. Oral preparations are poorly absorbed from the stomach, so the preferred route of administration for more intensive treatment is intravenous. Schedules are shown in Table 6.1.

8.2 Context of treatment

Bisphosphonates may be considered for patients with prostate cancer in a number of distinct situations: 1) For castration refractory metastatic prostate cancer, 2) With initial hormone therapy, either in localised disease to prevent/delay development of bone metastases, or as a component of systemic treatment of metastatic disease, 3) To reduce osteoporosis in patients on long term hormone deprivation or on corticosteroids.

8.3 Castration refractory prostate cancer

In 2002, Saad et al. reported a prospective randomized trial in patients with castration refractory metastatic prostate cancer which compared in three arms patients having zoledronic acid at 4 mg iv every 3 weeks or 8 mg iv every 3 weeks or placebo. Patients continued with hormone deprivation therapy or other anticancer therapies as indicated. There were just over 200 men in each arm of the study, the median age was 72–73 years and the primary endpoint of the study was development of a skeletal related event (SRE) such as pathological fracture, spinal cord compression, surgery or radiotherapy for bone pain or a change in anticancer treatment for bone pain. The higher dose of zoledronic acid was associated with renal damage and therefore during the study, those randomized to the 8 mg dosage had subsequently the dose reduced to 4 mg. Toxicities of the active treatment arms included anaemia, fever, oedema, fatigue, and myalgia. At 15 months, there were fewer SREs in men originally randomized to the 4 mg dosage than in those randomized to placebo (33% vs 44%, P = 0.02). However, the difference between those randomized to zoledronic acid at 8 mg and placebo was not significant. There were no differences in disease progression, performance status or quality of life scores among the group. Thus the use of zoledronic acid in this patient population must be judged by balancing the risk of toxicity, now known to also include jaw necrosis, with a quantitation of the benefit.

A Canadian trial evaluated intravenous clodronate in symptomatic men at 1500 mg every 3 weeks in conjunction with chemotherapy with mitoxantrone and prednisone. There was no significant difference in palliative benefit from that achieved by mitoxantrone and prednisone with placebo.

Two trials of pamidronate for the palliation of bone pain in men with metastatic prostate cancer have been subject to combined analysis. They included 378 patients with symptomatic bone metastases. Pamidronate at 90 mg every 3 weeks for 9 doses was compared with placebo and the primary endpoint was a change in pain score. There was no significant difference in pain score at 9 weeks, in morphine equivalent analgesia or in the risk of skeletal related events. A metaanalysis of trials assessing pain control and bisphosphonates suggested benefit at 4 weeks though this was lost by 3 months. The current guideline in the UK from the National Institute for Health and Clinical Excellence (NICE) (2008) recommended that 'bisphosphonates for pain relief may be considered for men with hormone-refractory prostate cancer when other treatments (including analgesics and palliative radiotherapy) have failed'.

Table 8.1 Bisphosphonate schedules assessed for metastatic prostate cancer

Drug	Route	Dose	Frequency
Zolodronate	iv	4 mg	3–4 weekly
Clodronate	po	520 mg	4 x per day
Pamidronate	iv	90 mg	3 weekly
Ibandronate	iv	6 mg	3–4 weekly daily
	po	60 mg	

Thus, although bisphosphonates have an established role in the treatment of patients with bone metastases from breast cancer and with bone lesions from multiple myeloma, the situation with castration refractory prostate cancer is less clear cut in terms of therapeutic ratio, possibly because these metastases are primarily osteoblastic. Current NICE guidance does not recommend the use of bisphosphonates to 'prevent or reduce the complications of bone metastases in men with hormone refractory prostate cancer', but this advice contains the qualification that there is inconsistent evidence, from several randomized clinical trials, of the effectiveness of bisphosphonates in this setting.

8.4 **Bisphosphonates with initial hormone therapy**

The UK Medical Research Council conducted a trial (PR05) in patients with known prostate cancer bone metastases who were starting or responding to hormonal therapy. The randomization was between oral sodium clodronate at a dose of 2080 mg per day vs placebo tablets. The primary endpoint was symptomatic bone progression or death from prostate cancer. The median time to symptomatic progression increased from 19 months to 24 months (p = 0.09). After a median follow up of 11.5 years estimated overall 5 and 10 year survival rates were 21% and 9% with placebo and 30% and 17% with clodronate (H.R 0.77, p = 0.03). This was the first trial suggesting an overall survival benefit with bisphosphonate treatment in prostate cancer but it is important to note the result was not replicated in men without metastases treated in the parallel Medical Research Council Trial (PR04) where there was no evidence of any benefit. A similar study using zoledronic acid at 4 mg iv every 4 weeks vs placebo was halted after recruitment of 398 subjects, because of a lower than expected event rate. In those who had entered the study, there was no difference in time to first bone metastases comparing the two groups.

8.5 **Trials currently in progress**

There remains considerable clinical interest internationally in developing the role in prostate cancer of particularly the more potent bisphosphonates such as zoledronic acid. Randomized controlled trials include the European Association of Urology 'ZEUS' trial, and the Trans Tasman Radiation Oncology Group 'RADAR' trial in men presenting with locally advanced disease, the Cancer and Leukaemia Group B trial with initial hormone therapy in men with metastatic disease, and in the UK, the 'STAMPEDE' trial, assessing a variety of additional treatments with initial hormone therapy of either locally advanced or metastatic disease, including one arm with zoledronic acid, one with both zoledronic acid and celecoxib and one with both zoledronic acid and docetaxel.

8.6 **Bisphosphonates for osteoporosis**

Studies have shown that bisphosphonates at lower dose intensities are effective in preventing bone mineral loss and fractures associated with the low hormone state. This is clearly relevant to patients having long term hormone deprivation or long term corticosteroid therapy for prostate cancer. Alendronate (oral, weekly) or intravenous pamidronate, zoledronic acid or risedronate given 3–12 monthly have been shown to both prevent bone density loss or improve established osteoporosis. For example, a placebo-controlled trial in 2,127 patients who had just suffered a hip fracture showed significant benefit of a single annual infusion of zoledronic acid at a dose of 5 mg, with reduction of the rate of further fracture. No national guidelines for osteoporosis screening or treatment have yet been established.

8.7 **Toxicity**

Bisphosphonates have the capacity for renal damage and renal function and serum calcium should be monitored in those treated regularly. Systemic effects such as anaemia, fever, fatigue and myalgia are known side effects but a further problem that has been identified is osteonecrosis of mandibular and maxillary bone which appears to be a particular risk in those with poor dental hygiene or those having dental procedures while on bisphosphonate therapy. The risk is time-related and an analysis of 252 patients treated with bisphosphonates show a cumulative hazard of about 0.1 at 3 years rising to 0.2 at about 6 years. It is important that patients have dental screening before initiating long term bisphosphonate therapy.

Further reading

Loberg et al. (2005). Pathogenesis and treatment of prostate cancer bone metastases: targeting the lethal phenotype. *J Clin Oncol*, **23**, 8232–41.

Dearnaley et al. (2003). A double blind placebo controlled randomised trial of oral sodium clodronate for metastatic prostate cancer. *J Natl Cancer Inst*, **95**, 1300–11.

Saad et al. (2002). A randomized placebo-controlled trial of zoledronic acid in patients with hormone-refractory metastatic prostate cancer. *J Natl Cancer Inst*, **94**, 1458–68.

Small *et al.* (2003). Combined analysis of two multicenter randomized studies of pamidronate disodium for the palliation of bone pain in men with metastatic prostate cancer *J Clin Oncol*, **21**, 4277–84.

Shahinian *et al.* (2005). Risk of fracture after androgen deprivation for prostate cancer. *N Engl J Med*, **352**, 154–64.

Lyles *et al.* (2007). Zoledronic acid and clinical fractures and mortality after hip fractures. *N Engl J Med*, **357**, 1799–1809.

Bamias et al. (2005). Osteonecrosis of the jaw in cancer after treatment with bisphosphonates: incidence and risk factors. *J Clin Oncol*, **23**, 8580–7.

Chapter 9

Systemic isotope therapy of bone metastasis

Christopher C Parker

Key points

- Sr-89 or Sm-153 improve pain control and quality of life, and delay the onset of new bone pain in men with CRPC and bone metastases
- Sr-89 or Sm-153 are recommended as standard of care in current prostate cancer treatment guidelines
- Sr-89 or Sm-153 may have a useful role not just in pain relief, but also in the prevention of skeletal-related events
- Sr-89 and Sm-153 can cause haematologic toxicity, and should not normally be used in men who are likely to require cytotoxic chemotherapy
- Ra-223 is a bone seeking alpha emitter, which may offer a better therapeutic ratio, with less myelosuppression.

9.1 The clinical problem of bone metastases

Castration-refractory prostate cancer (CRPC) has a propensity for bone marrow involvement. As many as 9 out of 10 men with advanced disease may have bone metastases, and often the bony skeleton will be the only known site of disease, with a lack of soft tissue or visceral disease on routine imaging. Characteristically, bone metastases from prostate cancer appear sclerotic on plain radiographs, and as areas of increased uptake on bone scintigraphy (Figure 9.1). When bone metastases become symptomatic, they may lead to bone pain, spinal cord or root compression, pathological fracture, and pancytopenia. These problems, sometimes referred to collectively as skeletal-related events, can cause major disability. Since the course of CRPC is often protracted over months or years, the morbidity due to bone metastases may be long-lasting.

The management of patients with bone metastases from prostate cancer includes hormone therapy, chemotherapy, analgesia, radiotherapy, and, on occasions, surgery for fixation of fractures or as an alternative to radiotherapy for spinal cord decompression. External beam radiotherapy is commonly used for men with bone pain that is resistant to simple analgesia, and achieves pain relief in around 8 out of 10 cases. However, external beam radiotherapy is a local treatment, whereas bone metastases in prostate cancer are typically multifocal. Hence there is a rationale for bone-seeking radioisotopes that can deliver radiotherapy to metastases throughout the skeleton.

Figure 9.1 Bone scan demonstrating multiple areas of increase uptake from prostate cancer metastases

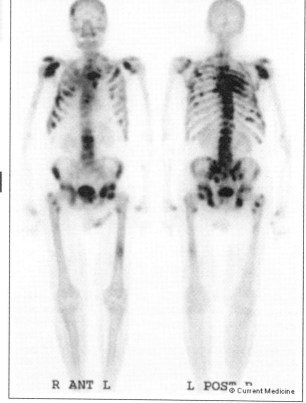

9.2 Characteristics of bone-seeking radio-isotopes

Bone seeking-radionuclides such as strontium-89 (^{89}Sr), samarium-153 ethylenediaminetetramethylene phosphonic acid (^{153}Sm-EDTMP), and rhenium-188-hydroxyethylene diphosphonate (^{188}Re-HEDP) have been used for many years in the treatment of men with bone metastases from prostate cancer. They are given by intravenous injection, and selectively target the osteoblastic reaction associated with bone metastases in one of two ways. Strontium, which is immediately below calcium in the periodic table, is metabolized in the same way as calcium, and deposited in the bone matrix. Other isotopes, such as rhenium-186 and samarium-153, which do not themselves have specificity for bone, are bound to a bisphosphonate (e.g. ^{186}Re-HEDP and ^{153}Sm-EDTMP).

9.2.1 Strontium-89

When strontium-89 is given intravenously, it is preferentially deposited in bone metastases rather than normal bone, at a ratio of around 10:1. It is bound in the bone for approximately 100 days, and delivers beta-irradiation with a half-life of 50 days. It is usually given at a standard administered activity of 150 MBq. The beta-radiation has a maximum range in tissue of a few millimetres, and the treated patient poses no direct radiation risk to others. Excretion is predominantly renal, and men may be advised not to use urinals for the first week after treatment. Men who are incontinent of urine may receive strontium-89 provided that they are catheterized.

9.2.2 Samarium-153

Samarium-153 has been used in the treatment of men with metastatic prostate cancer for over 10 years. It accumulates in bone metastases, rather than normal bone, at a ratio of around 5:1, and is a beta-emitter. The half-life of samarium-153 is considerably shorter than that of strontium-89, and so the duration of pain relief, and of myelosuppression, should also be shorter. Unlike, strontium-89, samarium-153 also emits gamma radiation, and this can be detected using a gamma camera to image the distribution of the radio-isotope.

9.2.3 Rhenium-188

Although rhenium-188 has been studied less extensively than strontium-89 and samarium-153, it is notable for its ease of production. A tungsten-188 generator (known as a rhenium 'cow') provides a ready source of rhenium-188 available for use whenever it is needed. The generator costs around £10,000, but then provides a long-lasting source of rhenium-188, that can be linked to HEDP and used for treatment.

The physical properties of these radioisotopes are summarized in Table 9.1.

Table 9.1 Characteristics of bone-seeking radioisotopes

Radionuclide	Carrier	Half-life (days)	Beta-max energy (MeV)	Max range in tissue (mm)	Gamma photon energy (keV)
Strontium 89	-	50.5	1.46	6.7	0
Samarium 153	EDTMP	1.95	0.8	3.4	103
Rhenium 188	HEDP	0.7	2.12	11.0	155

EDTMP–ethylenediaminetetramethylene phosphonic acid; HEDP–hydroxyethylene diphosphonate.

9.3 Evidence for efficacy

Two small randomized controlled trials in men with CRPC have shown that a single treatment with strontium-89 is significantly more effective than placebo in terms of pain control. One of these trials also found that strontium significantly prolonged overall survival. However, these studies did not compare strontium with the standard of care for men with painful bone metastases, namely external beam radiotherapy.

The clinical utility of strontium-89 was established by two pivotal randomized controlled trials. The Canadian trial, reported by Porter et al. in 1993, randomized 126 men with bone pain from CRPC, all of whom received external beam radiotherapy, to either 400 MBq strontium-89 or placebo. The men allocated to strontium-89 showed significant benefits in terms of need for analgesia, new sites of pain, freedom from further external beam radiotherapy, quality of life and physical activity. For example, the median time to new external beam radiotherapy for pain at any skeletal site was 8.1 months v 4.6 months for strontium and placebo, respectively (p = 0.006).

The British trial randomized 284 patients with CRPC and painful bone metastases to receive either external beam radiotherapy or 200 MBq of strontium-89, and was reported by Quilty et al. in 1994. Pain relief at the index site was equivalent, but significantly fewer patients reported new site of pain after strontium-89 than after external beam radiotherapy (36% versus 58%, p < 0.05), and significantly fewer required additional external beam radiotherapy within 12 weeks (3% versus 25%, p < 0.01).

The role of samarium-153 has been studied in three randomised controlled trials that included men with CRPC. These trials demonstrated effective pain relief for samarium-153 in comparison with placebo. However, no trials have compared the efficacy of samarium with that of external beam radiotherapy. It is widely assumed that samarium-153 and strontium-89 have similar efficacy, but this has not been formally tested. It is apparent that the onset of pain relief is more rapid for men treated with samarium (5-10 days) than with strontium-89 (2–3 weeks). Conversely, the duration of pain relief may be longer with strontium-89. Re-treatment should be considered when pain recurs.

The only randomized trial of rhenium-188 in CRPC compared a single treatment versus two treatments, eight weeks apart. The trial included just 64 patients, but, intriguingly found an overall survival benefit for men randomized to two treatments (median survival 12 months versus 7 months, p = 0.04).

9.4 Toxicity

Pain flare is often the first adverse effect following treatment. Men may experience a temporary exacerbation of bone pain within the first week following treatment, that may persist for several days. There is some evidence to suggest that those men that do experience bone flare may subsequently get a better pain response.

The commonest form of toxicity is haematological, with anaemia, leucopaenia and thrombocytopaenia. These adverse events are common, occurring in up to 80% of treated patients, but are usually mild and recover spontaneously. For example, in the British randomized trial of strontium-89, that included over 200 patients, grade III/IV platelet toxicity occurred in 7% of patients, compared with 3% of those treated with radiotherapy, and grade III leucopaenia was seen in 3% versus 0%, respectively. The timing of the platelet nadir is around 6 weeks for strontium-89, and around 3–4 weeks for samarium-153. Men with CRPC often have anaemia and thrombocytopaenia from their disease. The use of strontium-89 or samarium-153 is usually restricted to patients with a pre-treatment platelet count > 100. Anaemia, in the absence of thrombocytopaenia, need not be an absolute contraindication to radio-isotope treatment. Indeed, treatment with strontium-89 can lead to an improvement in haemoglobin levels in patients who are anaemic as a result of bone marrow infiltration with prostate cancer. In the British randomized trial, there was a trend towards fewer blood transfusions in those patients randomised to strontium-89 rather than external beam radiotherapy (19% versus 23%).

The long-term effects of radio-isotope treatment on bone marrow function are uncertain. It is standard practice to use strontium-89 or samarium-153 after, rather than before, cytotoxic chemotherapy, given the concern that previous radio-isotope treatment could impair bone marrow reserve. There is also a theoretical risk of myelodysplasia as a late adverse event after radioisotope treatment, but, since the life-expectancy of men with advanced CRPC is usually less than two years, this is not a major consideration.

9.5 **Radiation protection**

Radioisotopes are usually given by a nuclear medicine physician. Secure intravenous access is important to prevent extravasation, which could lead to radiation toxicity to local tissues. Samarium-153 and rhenium-188 emit some gamma radiation, and patients should be treated in a lead-lined room to minimize the hazard. Beta-particles have only a short range in tissue and pose little risk to others. Departments using radio-isotopes need to have standard policies for their safe storage and administration, and for dealing with spillages.

Patients, and their relatives, should know that their blood and urine may pose a radiation hazard within the first 10 days after treatment. For example, patients should use a toilet rather than a urinal, should take care to avoid spilling urine, should flush the toilet twice, and wash their hands afterwards.

9.6 **Combined modality treatment**

Attempts have been made to enhance the effect of strontium-89 by using concomitant chemotherapy, as a radiosensitizer. Cisplatin in low dose has been shown to improve pain palliation in patients treated with strontium-89 in a randomized trial. In a trial of 70 patients with CRPC, overall pain relief occurred in 91% of patients receiving Strontium-89 + cisplatin compared to 63% of patients receiving Strontium-89 + placebo (P < 0.01). Significantly less bone disease progression was observed in the experimental arm (27% versus 64%), with no clinically significant difference in toxicity between the arms. This approach remains experimental.

An alternative approach is the sequential use of strontium-89 after chemotherapy. Seventy two patients with CRPC responding to chemotherapy were randomized to receive further doxorubicin chemotherapy with or without strontium-89. There was a statistically significant improvement in median survival for the group receiving strontium-89 (28 months versus 17 months (p=0.0014). This strategy is now being tested in the TRAPEZE trial, which aims to recruit over 1,000 patients.

9.7 **Future developments**

The established radio-isotopes all emit beta particles (electrons) that produce relatively low energy radiation with a track length in tissues of up to several millimetres. In contrast, radium-223 is an alpha-emitter that localises to bone metastases because it is metabolized in the same way as calcium. Radium-223 produces high-linear energy transfer (LET) alpha radiation with a range of < 100 micrometres. In comparison with beta-emitters, a bone-seeking alpha-emitter might have a greater anti-tumour effect, by virtue of the densely ionizing high-LET radiation, but with relative sparing of the bone marrow due to the short track length. In a randomized, double blind, placebo controlled study of 64 patients with CRPC, radium-223 was extremely well tolerated, with little or no haematologic toxicity, and demonstrated encouraging evidence of efficacy. The excellent toxicity profile means that radium-223 can be given regularly. The ALSYMPCA trial will compare radium-223 versus placebo in 750 patients with CRPC who will receive 6 treatments over 6 months in addition to their standard care.

9.8 **Conclusions**

Radio-isotopes such as strontium-89 and samarium-153 have an important role in the treatment of men with bone metastases from CRPC. There is good evidence that they improve pain control, delay the development of new sites of pain, and reduce the need for external beam radiotherapy. There is some evidence, although less compelling, that they also improve quality of life and overall survival. It is interesting to compare the evidence supporting the use of radio-isotopes in CRPC with that regarding the use of bisphosphonates. Bisphosphonates have been shown to prevent skeletal related events, such as the need for external beam radiotherapy, but the magnitude of the effect is less than for radioisotopes. Furthermore, unlike strontium-89, current evidence suggests that bisphosphonates do not have a beneficial effect on quality of life.

There are no good data on the level of usage of radio-isotopes in the treatment of CRPC, but it seems likely that they are not used as widely as they should be. At present, radio-isotope treatment tends to be reserved for men with intractable bone pain that has not responded to either analgesia or external beam radiotherapy, or for men with multi-focal pain that is not amenable to external beam treatment. There is a rationale for using strontium-89 or samarium-153 earlier, in men with progressive CRPC and minimally symptomatic bone metastases. The aim of such treatment would be not just to achieve pain control, but also to prevent new sites of pain, to reduce the need for subsequent external beam radiotherapy, and possibly to improve quality of life and overall survival.

It is difficult to perform high quality clinical trials of radio-isotopes in CRPC, not least because the patient population tends to have a poor performance status, making compliance with treatment and outcome assessments difficult. Not surprisingly, there are many unanswered questions regarding the optimum use of radio-isotopes. It is not clear which patients are most likely to benefit, whether one radio-isotope is better than another, and how their use should be combined with that of other standard treatments such as chemotherapy. A high priority should be given to the ongoing phase III trials of radio-isotopes, such as TRAPEZE and ALSYMPCA. Patients with bone metastases from CRPC who are not in clinical trials should be considered for treatment with either strontium-89 or samarium-153.

Further reading

Finlay IG, Mason MD, Shelley M. Radioisotopes for the palliation of metastatic bone cancer: a systematic review (2005). *Lancet Oncol*, **6**, 392–400.

Porter AT, McEwan AJ, Powe JE, Reid R, McGowan DG, Lukka H, *et al.* (1993) Results of a randomized phase-III trial to evaluate the efficacy of strontium-89 adjuvant to local field external beam irradiation in the management of endocrine resistant metastatic prostate cancer. *Int J Radiat Oncol Biol Phys*, **25**(5), 805–13.

Quilty PM, Kirk D, Bolger JJ, Dearnaley DP, Lewington VJ, Mason MD, *et al.* (1994) A comparison of the palliative effects of strontium-89 and external beam radiotherapy in metastatic prostate cancer. *Radiother Oncol*, **31**(1), 33–40.

Chapter 10

Biological targets and new drug development for prostate cancer

Shahneen Sandhu and Johann DeBono

> **Key points**
>
> - Androgen receptor (AR) signalling is usually necessary for the development and progression of prostate cancer
> - Androgen depletion is the mainstay of treatment for advanced prostate cancer but responses can be short-lived
> - AR-signalling frequently remains intact as prostate cancer evolves from androgen sensitive to castration resistant disease (CRPC)
> - A number of mechanisms may facilitate AR reactivation, including AR overexpression, AR mutation leading to promiscuous ligand binding or constitutive activation, adrenal and intratumoral androgen synthesis, and activated signal transduction pathways
> - The AR signalling pathway remains a rational therapeutic target in CRPC.

10.1 Introduction

Androgen deprivation therapy (ADT) results in effective control of metastatic prostate cancer for a period of several years, but these patients inevitably progress as the cancer acquires resistance through modulation of androgen receptor (AR) signalling. Secondary hormonal therapy responses are at best short-lived. What has been commonly known as hormone resistant prostate cancer, but better described as castration resistant prostate cancer (CRPC), remains the second commonest cause of male cancer mortality after lung cancer, with a median survival of approximately 12 months after docetaxel treatment. The tubulin binding drug, docetaxel, offers effective palliation but only a modest survival advantage of 2–3 months. Better treatments that offer a survival advantage in patients with CRPC remain an unmet medical need.

The identification of aberrant signalling pathways implicated in prostate cancer progression and the greater appreciation of the underlying molecular basis for castration resistance has established a new paradigm for rationally-designed targeted agents. This chapter will outline the therapeutic targets in clinical development and will consider the challenges for future drug development for this disease.

10.2 **The androgen receptor: structure and function**

The AR is a member of the steroid hormone receptor family and functions as a ligand-activated nuclear transcription factor. Inactive AR is localized to the cytoplasm where it is bound to heat shock proteins (HSPs) which stabilize its structural conformation to facilitate ligand binding. AR undergoes conformational change upon ligand binding, dissociates from HSPs, and translocates into the nucleus where it binds to androgen response elements, recruiting other proteins and forming complexes to modulate the transcription of target genes. These recruited co-activator and co-repressor proteins facilitate or silence gene transcription and can themselves be regulated by post-translational modification through methylation, acetylation and phosphorylation.

10.3 **Castration-resistant phenotypes and molecular targets**

AR signalling is implicated in the development of prostate cancer and frequently remains critical as the tumour becomes castration resistant. Castration-resistant phenotypes (CRPC) can emerge as a consequence of: (1) AR signalling reactivation despite the systemic castrate state in a ligand dependent or ligand independent fashion, (2) the development of AR-independent tumorgenic pathways through other signalling pathways and (3) enhanced regulatory protiens which confer antiapoptotic activity.

The AR can acquire hypersensitivity to low levels of androgen through activating gene mutations, amplifications, overexpression, and enhancement of transcriptional coactivator function and is then able to circumvent circulating castrate androgen levels to maintain androgen mediated AR signalling. Additionally, cellular adaptation in the androgen-suppressed environment is postulated to result from enhanced adrenal and local intracrine synthesis of testosterone and 5-dihydrotestosterone (DHT) from precursor steroids, providing a sustained intratumoral source of androgens to drive ongoing AR signalling. Hence AR remains an important therapeutic target.

Activating AR gene mutations may either enhance AR sensitivity or diminish ligand specificity, resulting in AR activation with low androgen levels or with a promiscuous range of other steroids and even AR antagonists. Mutant AR studied in the context of anti-androgen withdrawal response indicates that mutations in the hormone binding domain can have paradoxical AR agonist activity. AR mutations that lack the ligand binding domain and are constitutively active have also been described. Ligand–independent AR activation may result from upregulation of key growth and survival kinase signalling cascades such as the insulin growth factor-1 receptor axis, the phosphoinositide 3-kinase (PI3K) pathway, and the epidermal growth factor receptor family. Cross talk between the AR and collateral pathways such as Src signalling may also result in nongenomic AR activation. Src inhibitors can reduce cancer cell proliferation, invasion and metastasis. Overexpression of antiapoptotic proteins such as bcl-2 and survivin has also been implicated as a potentially important and AR independent mechanism of resistance.

10.4 The development of targeted treatment for prostate cancer

The key to rational targeted agent design is the characterization of abberant genetic and molecular pathways that drive the pathogenesis and progression of the disease. Once the dominant dysregulated signalling pathway is defined, a drug can be designed to target this pathway. A perfect example of this is the Philadelphia chromosome t(9;22) (q34;q11) resulting in the BCR-ABL fusion gene which is implicated in the pathogenesis of chronic myeloid leukemia (CML). The identification of this single 'druggable' pathway provides a point of weakness that can be therapeutically exploited as is the case with Imatinib mesylate, an inhibitor of the BCR-ABL tyrosine kinase which has revolutionized threatment of CML. Most solid tumours however have multiple parallel and intertwined signalling pathways that allow the tumour to circumvent blockade at one site by collateral signalling, attesting to the need for a combined approach of targeting interacting growth pathways concurrently.

In CRPC, several druggable mechanisms that allow continued AR signalling in the castrate enviroment have been postulated, providing the impetus for more effective abrogation of these pathways, as well as less specific targets (Figure 10.1). These strategies include more effective anti-androgens to directly block AR ligand binding; inhibitors of CYP17 to impede both *de novo* intracrine tumour-generated AR ligands as well as intratumoral conversion of adrenal steroids to more active androgenic metabolites; inhibitors of HSP90 to destabilize the AR; inhibitors of histone deacetylases which can govern AR-target

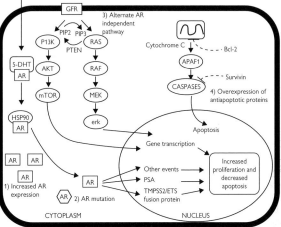

Figure 10.1 Proposed mechanisms of androgen resistance and biological targets in castration resistant prostate cancer

Mechanisms of androgen resistance:
1. AR hypersensitivity by amplification, over expression or modulation in corepressor/coactivator function
2. AR mutations resulting in nonandrogenic ligand binging and activation
3. Ligand independent down stream activation of AR signalling
4. Upregulation of antiapoptotic proteins

Novel therapeutic targets:
1. Adrenal and intratumoral steroid synthesis
2. Conversion from testosterone to the more potent metabolite 5-DHT
3. AR signalling
4. Growth factor receptors (GFR), PTEN (phosphate and tensin homolog), PI3K (phosphatidylinositide 3-OH kinase) signalling
5. Angiogenesis
6. Apoptosis

transcription and tyrosine kinase inhibitors which block other alternative stimulatory pathways (Table 10.1). The identification of the ETS gene fusion proteins (translocations) such as TMPRSS2-ERG suggests that directly targeting the activity of these potent oncogenes will be an important future area for research. Finally, the presence of estrogen receptor **(ERα and ERβ) response and repressor elements suggest that targeting estrogens** may also play a more important role in prostate cancer therapy in the future.

Table 10.1 Targeted agents under evaluation for CRPC

Agent	Target	Biological effect
Abiraterone acetate	17α hydroxylase/ C17,20-lyase	Supression of adrenal and de nova androgen synthesis

Anti-androgens
  MDV-3100
  BMS-641988
	Androgen Receptor	Prevents nuclear translocation and DNA binding of AR & prevents androgen binding to the receptor

5 alpha-reductase inhibitors Dutasteride	5 alpha-reductase	Blocks the conversion from testosterone to dihydrotestosterone
HSP-90 inhibitors 17-AAG	HSP90	Destabilization and destruction of the AR
HDAC inhibitors Depsipeptide (FK288) LBH589 SAHA	HDAC	Downregulates AR and AR targeted genes

Vitamin D analogues
  DN-101
  EB1089
	Vitamin D Receptor	VDR mediated antiproliferative effects

IGFI-R targeting monoclonal antibodies CP-751871 IMC-A12	IGFI-R	Inhibits IGFI-R signalling axis
PI3 kinase inhibitors BEZ235 GDC0941	PI3 kinase	Inhibits the PI3 kinase signalling axis
mTOR inhibitors CC1-799 RAD001	mTOR	Inhibition of downstream effects of the PI3/AKT pathway
Antiangiogenics Bevacizumab AZD2171 Sorafenib Thalidomide & analogues	 VEGF VEGFR VEGFR bFGF, VEGF, TNF-alpha	Prevents neovascularisation & enhanced delivery of cytotoxics to the tumour
ET-A Atrasentan Zibotentan	Endothelin A receptor	Inhibits angiogenesis, proliferation, invasion and metastasis
SRC inhibitors Dasatinib Saracatinib	Scr/abl	Inhibits angiogenesis, proliferation, migration and invasion

10.5 **Targeting AR signalling**

10.5.1 **Inhibiting adrenal and intratumoral steroid synthesis**

ADT does not achieve an androgen-free intratumural environment. Residual adrenal gland derived and de-novo intratumoral androgen biosynthesis may be sufficiently unregulated to promote persistent AR signalling. CYP17 is a key enzyme in this process. Ketoconazole, an imidazole anti-fungal agent is a weak non-specific inhibitor of several cytochrome P450 enzymes including CYP17. A third of patients who progress on anti-androgens have short-lived PSA responses to keto-conazole. This agent is often, however, poorly tolerated due to constitutional side effects and may interfere with the metabolism of other drugs. Moreover, it is not able to adequately suppress CYP17, with rising androgenic steroid levels reported at progression during ketoconazole therapy.

Abiraterone acetate (AA) is an orally bioavalable potent, selective and irreversible inhibitor of CYP17 with 17α-hydroxylase/C17, 20-lyase activity. It inhibits the two key catalytic reactions involved in the synthesis of androgenic steroids: 17α-hydroxylation of preg-nenolone and progesterone and the subsequent conversion of 17-hydroxypregnenelone and 17-hydroxyprogesterone to androgens, DHEA and androstenedione. Preclinical and clinical studies have confirmed effective inhibition of CYP17 with suppressed androgenic steroid synthesis downstream of CYP17 (DHEA, androstenedione and testosterone) and a corresponding rise in steroids upstream of CYP17 (progesterone, 11-deoxycorticosterone (DOC), 18-hydroxy-progesterone, and corticosterone) secondary to increased ACTH levels. Corticosterone and 11-deoxycorticosterone (DOC) are min-eralcorticoids with sufficient glucocorticoid activity to avoid adrenal insuffiency. As descrbed for congenital CYP17 deficiency, these excess upstream mineralcorticoids can however give rise to a syndrome characterized by fluid retention, hypertension and hypokalaemia. This can be easily managed with the mineralocorticoid receptor antago-nist, eplerenone and potassium supplementation or alternatively small dose of steroids used in conjunction with AA suffices to decrease ACTH levels.

The first phase I study of AA in patients with CRPC confirmed safety and established the recommended phase II/III dose at 1000mg daily. AA was well tolerated with no dose limiting toxicities. AA treatment resulted in decline in PSA, reduction in circulating tumour cell (CTC) levels, radiological responses and symptomatic benefit in up to 70% of patients. Phase II studies have reported antitumour activity in castration-resistant, docetaxel-naive and docetaxel-treated prostate cancer patients who had progressed on multiple hormonal regiments with PSA response in between 52%–60% and durable RECIST response rates of 21%–26%.

One of the postulated mechanisms of resistance to single–agent AA may include increased steroid production upstream of CYP 17 blockade leading to ligands activating a promiscuous and/or mutated AR. Concurrent use of low dose exogenous steroids is effective at decreasing the steroid levels upstream of CYP17 by decreasing ACTH levels. This strategy has salvaged a number of patients who had PSA progression on AA alone and serves as the basis for the combination of AA with steroids to minimize mineralcorticoid syndrome and resistance development.

A multi-centre, double-blinded phase III study of abiraterone acetate plus prednisolone versus placebo plus prednisolone in patients post-docetaxel is ongoing. Further phase III evaluation of AA in the pre-docetaxel setting is planned.

10.5.2 **Antiantrogens**

Anti-androgens block AR signalling by two main mechanisms: direct blockade of androgen-AR binding and inhibition of the transcription of androgen-regulated genes via inhibition of nuclear co-activators, and recruitment of nuclear co-suppressors. Characterization of the crystal structure and binding mechanisms of AR has led to the design of novel AR antagonists with promising activity.

MDV3100 (Medivatin Inc.) is a small molecule antagonist which blocks AR signalling by preventing the nuclear translocation and DNA binding of AR. MDV3100 does not display agonist activity in the face of AR overexpression and is able to overcome the resistance of conventional anti-androgens. MDV3100 showed promising regression of hormone refractory LANCAP-AR cells in a dose dependant manner and is currently being evaluated in phase I/II dose-escalation study in chemotherapy naïve and treated patients. MDV3100 is reported to be well tolerated with PSA responses observed in a more than half of the chemotherapy-naïve and treated patients. Patient accrual at higher doses is ongoing.

VN/124-1 is a steroidal benzoazole compound 5 (3β-hydroxy-17-(1H-benzimidazole-1-yl) androsta-5, 16-diene) with potent anti CYP17 and AR antagonistic activity. VN/124-1 has shown promising antiproliferation effects on bicalutamide-resistant prostate cancer cell lines (HP-LNCaP) that overexpressed ARs. The combination of VN/124-1 with everolimus or gefitinib showed enhanced antiproliferation effects on HP-LNCap cells compared to biclutamide. VN/124-1 merits further clinical development for the treatment of prostate cancer.

10.5.3 **5-reductase inhibitors**

Testosterone is converted to the more potent metabolite, dihydro-testosterone (DHT) by 5 alpha-reductase (type I and II). Dutasteride, a dual type I and II 5 alpha-reductase inhibitor resulted in an almost complete suppression of DHT and a marked increase in apoptosis of tumour cells in 46 men with T1 /T2 tumours following 6–10 weeks of treatment. A phase I/II study of LY320236, a dual 5 alpha-reductase inhibitor in 51 patients with CRPC showed a 50% PSA response of 27%. The serum levels of testosterone, dihydrotestosterone, and androstenediol glucuronide remained unchanged during treatment but there was an increase in serum estradiol levels which could potentially account for the responses.

A phase II trial of the combination of ketoconazole, hydrocortisone and dutasteride in 51 patients with CRPC reported a PSA response rate of 53% and a median time to progression (TTP) of 13.7 months which far superior to the previously reported TTP for ketoconazole and hydrocortisone alone.

10.5.4 **Heat shock protein-90 inhibitors (HSP90)**

Heat shock protein 90 (HSP90) is a ubiquitous molecular chaperone that is integral to the assembly, stabilization, localization, and proteolytic degradation of a wide range of client proteins including key cell signalling molecules involved in oncogenesis such as AR, ERα, ERB-B2, BCR-ABL, B-RAF, AKT, c-Met, HIF, etc. Inhibition of HSP-90 leads to proteasome-mediated degradation of these client proteins and consequently modulation of multiple signal transduction pathways implicated in cancer growth such as the RAS-RAF-mitogen-activated protein kinase and phosphatidylinositol 3-kinase pathways. HSP-90 bound to inactive AR functions to maintain protein structural integrity and prevent AR degradation. This may be especially critical for mutated proteins. Overall, HSP-90 inhibition leads to AR degradation, which reduces AR expression and inhibits tumour growth. HSP-90 inhibition with 17-allylamino, 17-demethoxygeldanamycin (17-AAG), a geldanamycin analogue in prostate cancer xenografts caused a marked reduction in HER2, AR, and Akt expression and inhibited proliferation. Improved, orally bioavailable, HSP90 inhibitors are now being evaluated in early clinical trials.

10.5.5 **HDAC**

Deacetylases have been reported to be potentially important targets for prostate cancer drug development. The antitumour effect of HDAC inhibitors in prostate cancer may be secondary to (1) suppressed transcription and expression of AR and AR target genes such as TMPRSS2 and p21; (2) reduced HDAC dependent ETS gene transcriptional activity; (3) HDAC6 blockade leading to HSP-90 inhibition by deacetylation which destabilizes AR. Suberoylanilide hydroxamic acid (SAHA), a HDACi has shown dose dependant prostate tumour suppression in preclinical models and is approved for used in T-cell cutaneous lymphoma. FK228 (Depsipeptide) has shown modest antitumour activity in CRPC.

10.5.6 **Insulin-like growth factor**

Insulin-like growth factor 1 (IGF-1) and IGF-2 are stimulatory ligands for IGF-1R, a tyrosine kinase receptor implicated in prostate cancer progression and resistance. Ligand binding results in activation of the intracellular signalling cascade including the Ras/MAPK and PI3K/AKT pathways, which mediate cellular transformation, proliferation and anti-apoptosis. IGF-1R activation may elicit ligand independent AR downstream signalling, thus contributing to resistance development.

IGF-IR inhibition results in antiproliferative effects, potentiates cytotoxic therapies, in vivo and in vitro prostate xenograft models. Docetaxel combination clinical studies are now evaluating IGF-IR targeting monoclonal antibodies. Other strategies to target the IGF-1R signalling cascade includes using small molecule insulin receptor and IGFR-specific thyrosine kinase inhibitors or inhibiting down stream signalling proteins such as mTOR and AKT.

10.5.7 **PTEN and phosphoinositide 3-kinase signalling**

The PI3K/AKT/mTOR signalling pathway is a key regulatory pathway of many essential cellular functions such as protein synthesis, cell proliferation, growth, and survival. Dysregulated PI3/AKT/mTOR pathway is implicated in the pathogenesis and progression of prostate cancer. PTEN, a tumour suppressor gene negatively regulates the PI3/AKT/mTOR pathway. Loss of PTEN function, which is well described in advanced prostate cancer, activates PI3K/AKT/TORC signalling which may promote ligand-independent AR activation through cross-talk. This can give rise to androgen escape and the emergence of CRPC. There are multiple novel therapeutic agents in clinical development that target the various components of this important signalling pathway. The most promising include the PI3 kinase, AKT and TORC 1/2 inhibitors which are currently in Phase I clinical evaluation.

10.6 **Targeting antiapoptotic proteins**

Bcl-2, survivin and clusterin and other antiapoptotic proteins have been reported to confer resistance to therapy in advanced CRPC. The first agents to target these proteins were antisense therapeutics which may not have maximally blocked target function. Improved agents targeting these proteins are now undergoing clinical evaluation.

10.7 **Endothelin-A antagonism**

Endothelin-1 (ET-1) is a 21-amino-acid peptide that binds two receptors, ETA and ETB, each of which exerts distinct biological effects. Activation of the ETA receptor by ET-1 is thought to promote several processes involved in the progression of prostate cancer, including inhibition of apoptosis, promotion of angiogenesis and invasion, and changes in skeletal biology associated with bone metastasis. Atrasentan and Zibotentan are orally bioavailable ETA receptor antagonists. Atrasentan has been studied in two placebo-controlled randomized phase 3 trials in patients with metastatic and nonmetastatic CRPC. Decreases in bone alkaline phosphatase and rate of PSA rise were observed, however the primary end point of delaying disease progression was not met in either study. Zibotentan has been evaluated in a placebo-controlled randomized Phase II trial which did not result in a statistical difference in the primary endpoint of time to progression but showed a trend for improved overall survival in the treatment arms. Treatment with ETA receptor antagonist is reported to be well tolerated with the predominant side effects related to vasodilatation with peripheral oedema, rhinitis, and headache. Further phase III evaluation of these agents either alone or in combination with Docetaxel in CRPC patients is ongoing.

10.8 **Targeting angiogenesis**

Targeting angiogenesis is attractive as neovascularization is key for tumour growth and metastasis. Antiangiogenic agents have proven clinical efficacy in colorectal cancer, breast, lung and renal cancer and is now being extended to prostate cancer as well. Tumour progression is associated with up-regulation of pro-angiogenic factors, such as vascular endothelial growth factor (VEGF), basic fibroblast growth factors (BFGF) and platelet derived growth factors (PDGF), etc via an autocrine and paracrine fashion. Antiangiogenic agents enhance anticancer drug delivery to the tumour by reducing the intratumural hydrostatic pressure. Bevacizumab, a humanized murine monoclonal antibody against VEGF has been evaluated in two separate phase II studies in combination with docetaxel plus thalidomide or docetaxel plus estramustine with encouraging results. A phase III study (CALGB90401) of docetaxel with and without bevacizumab is ongoing and its results are expected in 2009.

Small molecule tyrosine kinase inhibitors of VEGF-R, FGF, PDGF etc such as sunitinib, sorafenib, and AZD2171 provides an alternative mode of inhibiting angiogenesis. Their evaluation in this disease is also ongoing.

10.9 **Conclusion**

Unravelling the molecular biology that underpins CRPC has resulted in the development of a wide range of rationally-designed therapeutic approaches with a renewed emphasis on blocking AR signalling. As these approaches evolve it is imperative to define suitable biomarkers to improve the odds of successful anticancer drug development for this disease. These are critical for patient selection where predictive biomarkers may be able to categorize different molecular types of prostate cancer as already described for breast cancer (ER+, HER2+ and triple negative). Prostate cancer inter-patient disease heterogeneity may indeed be the most important explanation for the many reported negative Phase III studies. Pharmacodynamic biomarkers for proof of principle studies to evaluate degree and duration of target modulation are also important. Biomarker studies may also help characterize resistance mechanisms. Intermediate ('surrogate') endpoint biomarkers that robustly associate with overall survival and may give an earlier readout of promising antitumor activity are also urgently required since PSA decrement algorithms are not reliable predictors of clinical benefit. Preliminary studies suggest that circulating tumour cell (CTC) counts merit evaluation for these biomarker studies. Finally, it remains to be seen if a multipronged rationally-targeted approach that blocks the feedback activation of several key pathways could result in a well-tolerated but synergistic therapeutic effect.

Further reading

Chen CD, Welsbie DS, Tran C, et al. (2004). Molecular determinants of resistance to antiandrogen therapy. Nat Med, **10**, 33–9.

Holzbeierlein J, Lal P, LaTulippe E, et al. (2004) Gene expression analysis of human prostate carcinoma during hormonal therapy identifies androgen-responsive genes and mechanisms of therapy resistance. Am J Pathol, **164**, 217–27.

Montgomery RB, Mostaghel EA, Vessella R, et al. (2008). Maintenance of intratumoral androgens in metastatic prostate cancer: a mechanism for castration-resistant tumour growth. Cancer Res, **68**, 4447–54.

Reid A, Attard G, Barrie E, et al. (2008). CYP 17 inhibition as a hormonal strategy for prostate cancer. Nature Clinical Practice Urology, **5**, 610–20.

Taplin M-E. (2008). Androgen receptor: role and novel therapeutic prospects in prostate cancer. Expert Rev. Anticancer Ther, 2008, **8**(9), 1495–1508.

Tomlins SA, Laxman B, Dhanasekaran SM, et al. (2007). Distinct classes of chromosomal rearrangements create oncogenic ETS gene fusions in prostate cancer. Nature, **448**, 595–9.

Tomlins SA, Rhodes DR, Perner S, et al. (2005). Recurrent fusion of TMPRSS2 and ETS transcriptional factor genes in prostate cancer. Science, **310**, 644–8.

Index

U

V

W

Z

WITHDRAWN